The
LYONS
Lifestyle

The LYONS Lifestyle

THE SEVEN HARDEST (AND EASIEST) STEPS TO A HEALTHY BODY

M. Frank Lyons II, M.D.

WESTBOW
P R E S S°
A DIVISION OF THOMAS NELSON
& ZONDERVAN

WestBow Press books may be ordered through booksellers or by contacting:

WestBow Press
A Division of Thomas Nelson & Zondervan
1663 Liberty Drive
Bloomington, IN 47403
www.westbowpress.com
1 (866) 928-1240

ISBN: 978-1-5127-4027-1 (sc)
ISBN: 978-1-5127-4028-8 (hc)
ISBN: 978-1-5127-4026-4 (e)

Library of Congress Control Number: 2016906856

Print information available on the last page.

WestBow Press rev. date: 6/14/2016

DEDICATION

So often my patients have asked me to continue to research and write that I have now written this, my third book, to try to provide them with a tool that can help them with their nutritional health. I dedicate it to my patients and the millions of Americans who suffer maladies directly related to the nutritional disaster that has occurred across this land. My hope and prayer are that this book will serve as a guide to help each of us develop a nutritional plan that will truly improve our health.

ACKNOWLEDGMENTS

I want to thank my patients for their patience as I prepared this book for publication. Without their constant questioning of their nutritional health issues, I wouldn't have had the impetus to finish this project. They also prompted me with many questions that became discrete chapters in this manuscript.

My many thanks are poured out to the reviewers of this manuscript: Dr. Michael Kimmey, Dr. Glenn Deyo, and his wife, Ann. Their insightful comments strengthened the text and topics I covered.

My heartfelt thanks and appreciation go to Bob Steenrod. He spent countless hours helping me edit this book and prompted me with numerous suggestions to improve the final product. He has been such an amazing friend and supporter throughout this project.

I also want to thank my spouse, Clare, for tolerating me during these many months of discussing, writing, rewriting, editing, and finishing the manuscript. Without her constant support, this project wouldn't have been completed.

Finally, I'm the product of God's sculpting my existence and knowledge. Without Him, I would be lost and am forever grateful for His many blessings heaped on me. To Him I give all the glory and honor for the completion of this book.

The Improvement of Understanding
Is for Two ends: First, our own Increase of Knowledge;
Secondly, to enable us to Deliver that Knowledge to Others.
John Locke

CONTENTS

INTRODUCTION

All truths are easy to understand once they are
discovered: the point is to discover them.
Galileo Galilei

America has dramatically changed over the past sixty years. Many
scientific developments have perpetuated those changes. Some
advancements, such as space travel, computer technology, cell phones,
the World Wide Web, and sequencing of the human genome (to name
a few), have led to an expansion of knowledge that is faster than at
any time in history. The consequences of this newfound information
have been both good and bad. While advances of these technologies
have allowed us to learn faster and be more connected with each other,
they also helped foreigners plan, facilitate, and execute a multifaceted
bombing of America on September 11, 2001.

In the same era, other less dramatic changes also occurred in the
area of nutrition that led to good and bad outcomes. The introduction
of trans fats into the Western diet in the twentieth century allowed
processed food to be better preserved and retain a longer shelf life in
the grocery store. Unfortunately, this manufactured fat is now directly
linked to heart disease and many cancers.

Genetically engineered (GE) wheat is another example of a scientific
advancement that has massively increased the crop yield of wheat. This

has produced large supplies of this grain for the entire world, but at the same time the amount of gluten found in wheat increased nearly one thousand fold. Human exposure to this protein (gluten) has caused an explosion of celiac disease and other gastrointestinal problems in the decades following incorporation of GE wheat into our food supply.

The development of high-fructose corn syrup (HFCS) in the 1970s was another step forward for the food industry that led to an abundance of inexpensive sweeteners. This change brought down the price of sugar, sweetened food, and beverage products. At the same time, rapid expansion of jet airplane travel allowed fresh fruits from around the world to be placed in our grocery stores year round. The subsequent eight-fold increase in our consumption of fructose from HFCS, fruits, honey and juices led to metabolic syndrome, obesity, fatty liver, and other unintended harmful outcomes to our health. We will explore all these issues later in this book so I won't define these terms here.

While the aforementioned changes in the food industry occurred, a growing number of women joined and remained in the American workforce. This change contributed to rapid expansion of the fast-food industry, the processed food industry, and the dining-out experience as a way for families to cope with less food preparation time at home. The shift in the US diet to prepared food brought on more sugar, trans fat, omega-6 fat, and carbohydrate consumption. The human body wasn't engineered to handle this massive surge in carbohydrate metabolism, and this change has resulted in an obesity epidemic affecting our entire population.

At the same time we increased our carbohydrate intake, several changes happened to the fat content of our diets. First was the mandatory pasteurization of milk. Cows were moved off the pastureland of America and placed on feedlots. Their food was changed from grass-based diets to corn and soybean diets. The transformation in the cows' diet changed the fat composition of the farm animals and dairy products. Grass-based diets are rich in omega-3 fats, the parent oils for normal neurological function and anti-inflammatory processes of the human body. We don't make these fats and must ingest them regularly to maintain these body functions. Most omega-3 fatty acids previously found in our diets disappeared in the early 1960s and have never been restored. We're now seeing the medical consequences of this change.

The alternative diet of corn and soy, which farm animals were put on, changed the fat content from omega-3 to omega-6 fats in these commodities. Omega-6 fat is the primary fat found in corn and soy products and vegetable oils. This fat is the parent oil for initiating the inflammatory reactions in our bodies. We need a small amount of omega-6 fat in our diets to be able to fight infections, heal wounds, and repair our bodies after heavy exercise. Unfortunately, our omega-6 fatty acid consumption has skyrocketed in the past sixty years due to the increased use of corn, soybeans, and other omega-6-rich vegetable oils in nearly all processed foods. The medical consequences have been terrible.

Increased food production through genetic engineering, the development of trans fats, and the production of high-fructose corn syrup have led to our ability to feed many more people at much lower costs. These and other changes, which I review in this book, have also wreaked havoc on our health at an unprecedented rate.

My message may sound dire; the medical consequences of these dietary changes are bad. However, all these changes can be reversed for anyone. You just need to understand what various food choices do to your body, and learn to make better choices to improve your health.

My purpose in writing this book is to explore the changes to our diets over the past several decades. I will help you understand the medical disasters that have occurred because of those changes. Finally, I will outline a plan to help you reverse or prevent some of those health issues. While it's impossible to reverse all effects of consuming trans fats for forty years, data reveal that it's never too late to modify our diets in the many areas I outline in this book.

In that vein, I have developed the "Lyons Lifestyle" to help you initiate a focused set of instructions that will bring the changes necessary to regain your nutritional health. This seven-point lifestyle plan includes the elimination of all manufactured trans fats from your diet, the increase of omega-3 fats, the decrease of omega-6 fats, the decrease of fructose intake, and a decrease in gluten and grain consumption. While you incorporate these changes in your diet, my advice is to monitor the metabolic changes that will occur with initial and then quarterly blood testing until your affected blood chemistry abnormalities have corrected. Additionally, I outline simple guidelines for exercise, weight reduction, and waistline management for a balanced lifestyle change you can sustain. I've been teaching this approach with ongoing modifications for the past two decades and have seen amazing medical improvements in thousands of my patients.

Prevention is more advantageous than treatment when it comes to our health. This book provides a road map to pursue both. Our dietary changes over the past sixty years have produced many preventable or reversible diseases many of us across America now find ourselves plagued with. These have caused the health care industry to explode in many directions. We now find ourselves needing many medications to treat elevated cholesterol and triglycerides, diabetes, high blood pressure, gout, and a myriad of inflammatory diseases, mental problems, and even dementia.

These disorders and their required medications could be dramatically reduced if we were to incorporate the Lyons Lifestyle into our daily lives. There would be far fewer hospitalizations and visits to our health care providers, decreased laboratory and diagnostic imaging requirements, and fewer joint replacements because of joint failure. There would also be far less medication consumption. The savings in money spent on health care; in time lost from productive life because of pain, suffering, and attending to health care needs; and on the need for nursing assistance at home, assisted living, or extended care facilities could be astronomical.

My hope is that this resource will help you develop a long-term plan to improve your health and that of your loved ones. It could also lead to substantial financial savings in the years to come and possibly prevent or reverse diseases. The Lyons Lifestyle is a tool for us to use to facilitate real health care reform in the years to come.

CHAPTER 1

Eliminate Trans Fats

It has become appallingly obvious that our
technology has exceeded our humanity.
Albert Einstein

Some scientific discoveries, whether by accident or design, have been observed and led to amazing changes in our world. When Louis Pasteur accidentally observed that fungi could suppress the growth of bacteria, the concept of antibiotics was born. While one could argue that the use of antibiotics has been excessive on many occasions, Pasteur's observation dramatically changed medicine forever. Likewise, the application of a chemical reaction to vegetable oil led to the production of trans fats.

At the beginning of the twentieth century, a German chemist, Wilhelm Normann, tried to produce a lubricant from vegetable oil. By design he developed "white" grease by superheating vegetable oil in a pressure cooker and adding a catalyst to the pressurized, hot oil. This step led to a change in the structure of the oil, which caused it to solidify at room temperature. Unfortunately, when heated, it quickly liquefied again and wasn't very useful as a lubricant.

The positive properties of these trans fats as a cooking oil were spectacular, however. This additive would enhance food flavor, improve the quality of food texture in pies and pastries, and function as a preservative when used in food preparation. The Proctor & Gamble Corporation quickly realized these benefits and purchased the patent for US production in 1909. Crisco was born, changing the food industry forever. At the time, most people lived on farms and used butterfat, lard, and tallow as their cooking fats; therefore, Crisco wasn't accepted in many households before World War II.

During the war millions of American women left home and entered the civilian war-machine-manufacturing workforce to support the Allied forces against Hitler's Nazi regime and the Axis powers of Japan and Italy. At the end of World War II, many of those women continued working outside the home. The consequences of this shift in the labor force led to an explosion of the fast-food industry and the rapid expansion of processed foods available on grocery store shelves. The transformation from saturated fats (also known as farm fats—butter, lard, and tallow) to trans fats occurred rapidly. There was a national butter shortage, since much of this commodity was supplied to military personnel, and margarine (loaded with trans fats) became a suitable substitute. Fast-food restaurants used trans fats to cook french fries and deep-fried meats. Meanwhile grocery store shelves became filled with food products preserved with trans fats. New cookbooks, such as Betty Crocker cookbooks, were published and contained recipes promoting the inclusion of trans fats.

At the same time trans fats were promoted in restaurants and grocery stores, there was a push to eliminate the traditional saturated farm fats from our diets. By 1960, the typical American diet had moved away from farm fats to trans fats and vegetable oils (omega-6 fats). While this change occurred, the health risks from trans fat consumption began to emerge.

Trans fats initially seemed to be harmless, but simple and beneficial trans fats caused a sudden increase in heart disease and many cancers across America. By 1958 some realized that trans fats were the cause of this epidemic of diseases. Dr. Ancel Keys, from the University of Minnesota, produced data for President Dwight Eisenhower that exposed this connection. This information was given to the Food and Drug Administration, but another fifty years passed before that agency started to take steps to warn the American people about the toxicity of trans fats. Coincidentally, Dr. Keys was the developer of K rations for the US military; they were also loaded with trans fats. He also worked tirelessly to remove saturated farm fats from the world's diet. Ironically, he also began to promote a "Mediterranean" diet as an alternative to our diets.

When the early data came out about the link between trans fats and heart disease in the late 1950s, a massive lobbying effort in Washington, DC turned the nation's focus away from trans fats. Instead, beef and eggs became the scapegoat. They were high in saturated fat and cholesterol. Nutrition academia and food industry scientists convinced the Food and Drug Administration that these two fats were the "true cause" of heart disease. America was immediately placed on a low-fat, high-carbohydrate diet that contained massive quantities of trans fats, and for the next forty years, the health of America spiraled into rapid decline. Numerous diseases, including heart disease, cancer, inflammatory and degenerative diseases, autoimmune disorders, diabetes, kidney failure, hypertension, fatty liver disease, and obesity now affect millions of unaware Americans. As you'll learn by the end of this book, trans fats weren't the only cause of this explosion of diseases, but they clearly led the pack.

The response of the federal government and big business was to treat the emerging diseases with newfound medications and surgeries rather than trying to stop the cause of our failing health. The rapid expansion of the pharmaceutical industry now accounts for hundreds of billions of dollars per year. While this growth has led to massive increases in the cost of health care, the federal government has done very little to stop the underlying cause of these diseases. A recent paper published in the *British Medical Journal* revealed that there is zero correlation between egg consumption and heart disease or stroke (see Rong, et al, BMJ, 3013). A thirty-year review of the world's medical studies demonstrates that consuming farm fats that contain saturated fats and cholesterol isn't the cause of heart disease and stroke, while trans fats, which do cause these diseases, continue to be consumed daily and damage our health.

In the early 1980s, Dr. Mary Enig and others tried to warn the country about the harmful effects of trans fats. She and a handful of dedicated scientists worked diligently to educate America. It wasn't until twenty years later that a national awareness began to grow. In the interim, the intense lobbying efforts of the manufactured trans fat industry and nutrition academia ostracized her and her colleagues, who exposed the dangers of trans fats, and much important research was defunded in the process. This resistance only delayed the truth about this deadly fat being better understood and led to the suffering and death of untold numbers of Americans who succumbed to heart disease, stroke, blood vessel disease, and cancers.

Cities and counties across the United States began to pass ordinances to restrict the use of trans fats in restaurants in the early 2000s. California, New York, and other locales have now totally forbidden the use of trans fats in restaurants, since massive amounts of scientific data overwhelmingly condemned the continued use of them. The federal government followed suit by mandating the inclusion of trans fat content on the food labels of processed foods. The Food and Drug Administration required the manufactured food industry to include the quantity of trans fats per serving. The problem with how they constructed the regulation is that they allowed the industry to label foods as zero grams of the trans fat per serving if the product contained less than five hundred milligrams (one half of a gram) per serving.

Well-documented studies now show that consuming as little as two hundred milligrams of trans fat per day is enough to change your cholesterol profile so you're at increased risk of developing heart disease. National data as of 2000 revealed that the average American consumed six grams of trans fats per day. This number had decreased from peak consumption of eight to ten grams or more per day in the 1980s. This information is very misleading to the average consumer, who is trying to eliminate trans fats from his or her diet. If you're unaware of a deceptive food label, you could easily consume several grams of trans fats per day, all the while believing you're improving your diet.

If dozens of articles and sixty years of rapidly rising heart disease aren't enough evidence for nutrition and government experts to make a "definitive" statement, I would point this out: We didn't just start eating eggs and meat from farm animals and drinking whole milk in the last half of the twentieth century. We didn't have heart problems in other periods of American history, and most of our ancestors consumed these food products daily all their lives.

We are told today that people are now living longer, but let's look at the age of those who participated in the Lewis and Clark expedition in 1804. If they didn't suffer an injury that resulted in infection or contracted an infectious disease, they lived into their eighties without the use of medications or surgeries (those entities didn't exist in any meaningful way as yet). Thomas Jefferson lived to be eighty-three years old, Benjamin Franklin lived to be eighty-four, and John Adams lived to be to ninety. All three had intact mental faculties, and none had any artificial joints, prescribed pharmaceuticals, or treatments of kidney dialysis. George Washington lived into his late sixties and died from a peritonsillar abscess, which would be an easily treated condition with antibiotics today. They all lived consuming "zero grams trans fats (per serving)."

Today many of our elderly suffer from dementia and live in extended-care facilities, all the while needing numerous medications to treat their chronic diseases. Many have undergone cancer treatment, have required artificial joint replacement, and are sustained by regular renal dialysis for kidney failure. Millions have suffered a stroke or heart attack, but are they living longer?

If we were to turn the clock back to a time before the introduction of trans fats but could still dramatically reduce childhood infections (vaccinations and antibiotics) and prevent death related to infections acquired during child birth, trauma, pneumonia, skin infections, and so forth, the survivors would actually live longer, healthier lives without trans fats. You would see, as I regularly witness, excellent health in those individuals in my medical practice, who are living into their nineties and hundreds. Because they lived in the era before trans fat consumption but benefitted from modern vaccinations, antibiotics, and surgeries, many require minimal medications to maintain their health.

The baby boomer generation suffers from more medical problems than any other generation in American history. The damaging effects of trans fat, omega-6 fat, and now metabolic syndrome from daily excess fructose and other carbohydrates (more on these subjects in later chapters) have ravaged them. During the baby boomers' sixty years of a trans-fat–rich diet, heart disease exploded across America. When I was a medical student in 1978, about three hundred thousand people died annually from cardiac arrest. That number is now over eight hundred thousand per year. Two partners (who have no family history of heart disease) in my gastroenterology practice have even suffered from premature heart disease (ages forty-eight and fifty-two).

Two hundred milligrams of trans fats per day isn't much at all. It is the equivalent of eating three Ritz crackers, having one piece of cake, consuming a bowl of certain ice creams, or enjoying a soft tortilla wrap, if any of these items contain trans fats. And many processed foods still contain trans fats. Many of us can easily consume many of these foodstuffs each day and be completely unaware. You might enjoy a large piece of birthday cake at a noon celebration at the office, cheese and crackers during Monday night football, or a taco on the way home. We're all unaware of trans fats' ubiquitous presence, let alone the amount that accumulates over an average day of meals and snacks. Increasing our risk of heart disease from eating trans fat foods is only part of the story. Trans fat consumption is now also linked to several types of cancers. These include lymphoma, breast cancer, prostate cancer, skin cancer, esophageal cancer, and colon cancer. There has been a massive increase in these types of cancers in America over the past several decades. When I was a kid, all these cancers were rare, and most of us were unaware of anyone suffering or dying from one of them. Minimal treatment existed at that time, since few people suffered from these devastating ailments.

Disorders can begin in utero as well. Recent data now show that we're also at increased risk of developing heart disease at a young age. It may be seen in future studies that some of these other diseases are a consequence of high trans fat consumption. Prepubescent exposure to trans fats has also now revealed adverse effects on young adults. Girls who have consumed excess trans fats in their youth place themselves at increased risk of developing breast cancer at a young age.

The incidence of breast cancer now affects nearly every family in America. Trans fats are the primary risk. We also see other cancers that were once rare. Malignant melanoma is now a common skin cancer. The rising frequency of this disease has occurred in spite of a massive education effort to encourage people to wear hats and sunglasses, and apply sunscreens to protect them from the damaging effects of the sun's rays to their skin. My first question to individuals and academia which fail to look at the causes of melanoma in any meaningful way while primarily focusing on new treatments for this and other malignancies is this: did the sun start shining in the 1960s? While I don't disagree that prevention of melanoma by protecting our skin is rational, I have never heard it said that we should stop eating trans fats to reduce that risk in the first place. Likewise, we should get mammograms, prostate specific antigen (PSA) blood tests, and colonoscopies to screen for the development of breast, prostate and colon cancer, respectively, but we're never warned to stop consuming the primary causative agent, trans fats. We should be.

Another phenomenon has exploded in America over the past few years: erectile dysfunction, or ED, as millions now know it. Low testosterone is now being seen in many adult males; we see a discussion about this problem every evening during many television shows. The National Institutes of Health performed a study in the 1980s, linking trans fat consumption to low testosterone. This evidence has led to the pharmaceutical use of testosterone rather than addressing the cause. ED now affects nearly 40 percent of men over the age of forty-five. While low testosterone can have more than one cause, prospective data clearly show that trans fat consumption causes low testosterone and abnormal sperm motility. If you visit websites about low testosterone, you don't read about preventive measures or a major cause, only therapies. What's even more disheartening is that we now hear legal advertisements seeking clients who have been treated with testosterone therapy and suffered complications from it. At the same time, we've seen no legal action directed at the trans fat food or vegetable oil industry for the health damage that has occurred from consuming their products.

As I was preparing to write this chapter, I reviewed the most recent guidelines from the American Heart Association at their website (http://www.heart.org). They advise "cutting back on foods containing partially hydrogenated vegetable oils to reduce trans fat in your diet" and to "use naturally occurring, unhydrogenated vegetable oils" in food preparation and consumption. The Food and Drug Administration, the US Department of Agriculture, the Department of Health and Human Services, as well as medical and nutrition organizations all recommend eating an overall low-fat, high-carbohydrate (up to fifteen servings per day) diet. I feel we need to question past advice and develop better guidelines that reintroduce saturated fats (farm fats, palm oil, or coconut oil) back into our diets, since our nutritional health guidelines are failing us.

I purchased the latest edition of *Harrison's Principles of Internal Medicine* in preparation for writing this book. My desire was to review what the most up-to-date medical primer had to say about the risks of trans fats to our health. This text, now in its eighteenth edition and considered a primary authority for internal medicine for over sixty years, doesn't contain a *single* reference to trans fats. I cannot explain the lack of any discussion, even when there are thousands of published articles in the medical literature and even though the Food and Drug Administration has discussed its removal from our food chain because of the damage it causes to human physiology. It amazes me that, from the time since the first edition of the most knowledgeable textbook in medicine appeared in 1958 to the present time, our medical students and physicians haven't been educated in any way concerning the science surrounding trans fats. If they are so deadly that they must be removed from our diets because of the damage they cause, the health care establishment should have included those damages in our medical education.

There are now over sixty publications showing that trans fat intake increases total cholesterol, raises LDL (bad) cholesterol, and lowers HDL (good) cholesterol. These parameters are indicators health care providers have followed for decades in their attempt to reduce our ever-increasing risk of heart disease, and they have been well recognized by the American Heart Association for decades. Additionally, when trans fats are replaced with consumption of saturated fats, thirteen studies demonstrate that these cholesterol abnormalities significantly improve. Yet the American Heart Association recommends only that we should consider lowering our saturated fat and trans fat intake and replace it with liquid vegetable oils. Vegetable oils are high in omega-6 fats, which induce inflammation. I will cover the problems related to this guideline and these pro-inflammatory fats in another chapter. Suffice it to say, the problem isn't saturated fat. Additionally, trans fats are a primary problem when it comes to heart disease.

We've consumed massive doses of trans fats in America for over sixty years, and now millions of Americans are suffering the metabolic consequences. There are eight hundred thousand heart-related deaths per year, two hundred thousand women diagnosed annually with breast cancer, two hundred thirty thousand new cases of prostate cancer each year, one hundred twenty-three thousand new cases of colon cancer per year, sixty thousand new cases of lymphoma diagnosed annually, and one hundred sixty thousand new diagnoses of malignant melanoma per year. While trans fat consumption isn't the only risk factor for these diseases, very little education about its importance is even discussed in academic circles; little is said about prevention by the avoidance of trans fats. Rather, our focus is on early detection and treatment once we've acquired these diseases.

When I first published my book *42 Days to a New Life* in 2007 about the damaging effects of trans fats and the ensuing imbalance of essential fats in our Western diet, the data was rapidly expanding in the medical literature to support their injurious effects.

I have continued to research this issue since 2007, and I'm amazed by the hidden data that is still surfacing. In 1957 an autopsy study demonstrated that trans fats lead to calcification inside our cells and It's accumulation throughout our bodies. When I was an internal medicine resident in the early 1980s, my colleagues and I often commented on calcium deposits scattered through veins (phleboliths) and other tissues when we reviewed x-rays of patients admitted to the hospital. At that time, nobody could tell us why those calcifications were deposited there, but in retrospect it's obvious that calcified trans fats were accumulating in my patients' tissues and blood vessels.

Data reveal that even among individuals who have regularly consumed trans fat, cholesterol blood profiles dramatically improve with reduction or elimination of these hydrogenated vegetable oils.

There isn't a great deal of information yet to know whether we can reduce the risk of developing cancer or reversing low testosterone and the like by reducing trans fat intake for those of us who've been consuming them for over sixty years, but we can clearly educate our children and grandchildren about these risks. Maybe they can be spared the diseases that now ravage baby boomers all across America.

I want to touch on one other issue related to trans fats. Consumption of trans fats raises our "bad" LDL cholesterol, lowers our "good" HDL cholesterol, and raises our serum triglycerides. These are all biomarkers for heart disease. When this information was solidified in a series of studies in the early 1990s, the vegetable hydrogenation plants, which Unilever Corporation operated, that produced trans fats were closed in 1992 all across the European Union, but the United States didn't follow suit. The largest manufacturer of margarine in Europe, Unilever Corporation, removed trans fats and converted to palm oil use.

We are now up to eight hundred thousand deaths per year and rising from heart disease. Beyond these tragic deaths, the costs related to heart surgery, heart stents, heart medications, cholesterol medications, loss of work productivity, and the like amount to hundreds of billions of dollars annually. Just the use of statin medications to lower our "bad" LDL cholesterol costs patients and their insurance carriers about $900 billion annually. Add the suffering by millions of people because of the loss of loved ones; you would think that more would be done to try to reverse this tragedy. Even if we could see only a small decrease in all these medical problems, that would truly be health care reform. While American health is suffering, the federal government, academic nutrition, and the food industry haven't been honest with us. Not only have trans fats not been removed from our food supply, but there hasn't been an honest effort to educate us about the dangers of trans fats.

The federal government has allowed the food industry to label food as "zero grams trans fat per serving" as long as it contains less than five hundred milligrams "per serving," ignoring the studies that show that two hundred milligrams per day is all that's needed to increase one's risk of developing heart disease. The food industry is culpable in this too.

Several published studies have revealed that consuming trans fats during pregnancy leads to low birth-weight babies. Girls of those moms are then at increased risk of developing breast cancer early in life. Breast cancer was once considered a disease of those in the late middle age to the elderly. Trans fat consumption is changing that demographic.

A recent statement by the Food and Drug Administration says that up to seven thousand lives might be saved annually with the elimination of trans fats. As a result, they are considering removing this fat from the food chain. Why it has taken so many decades to reach their decision is unclear, but their figures understate the problem. Removal of this manufactured fat in other countries has reduced heart disease by almost 40 percent in the ensuing decades. Do the math; that's 40 percent of eight hundred thousand or three hundred twenty thousand people, not seven thousand. We're talking about people's lives, not some glib government statistic. Their discussion doesn't include any of the other diseases directly linked to trans fats, such as breast cancer, colon cancer, malignant melanoma, lymphoma, prostate cancer, and so forth. The figure is much higher than reported.

Learn to look at the food label's ingredient section to see whether your food product contains hydrogenated or partially hydrogenated fats. If it does, put the item back on the shelf and look for an alternative product. Look for products made with unprocessed palm or coconut oil instead. They don't cause heart disease or cancer. Don't rely on the "trans fat" part of the label, since food manufacturers have learned to manipulate the federal government guidelines to get that "zero grams trans fat per serving" on their product labels.

Pearls

- Trans fats cause heart disease.
- Trans fats cause cancer.
- Eliminate all trans fats from your diet.

CHAPTER 2

Increase Omega-3 Fatty Acids

There are two mistakes one can make along the road
to truth; not going all the way, and not starting.
Buddha

What would you need to know to respond to a child's simple request
to take him or her fishing? First, you would need to know where
fish can be caught. You might also need to know what the Fish and
Game Department rules and licensing requirements are for fishing.
You would finally need a fishing pole, tackle, bait, and the like: all this
just to go fishing.

Likewise, what do you need to know to maintain nutritional
health? You need to learn that there are essential components in foods
your body needs to maintain itself. You need to drink water. You need
vitamins and minerals. You need to consume amino acids in the form
of high-quality protein. Finally, you need to consume fats: omega-3
and omega-6 fats.

Our bodies require these fats (omega-3, omega-6, and some saturated
fats as I will point out later) to enable our immune and nervous systems
to function properly. There are also more subtle functions they are
involved in, and I will touch on some of those a bit later. Regular intake

of these fats is essential to human health, since our bodies don't have the ability to manufacture them. More importantly, they are required in the right ratio of omega-3 and omega-6 fats to maintain the proper balance in our immune system, nervous system, and inflammatory and anti-inflammatory processes. If our bodies are in a balanced state, we should be ingesting a ratio of about two to one of omega-3 to omega-6 fats. The correct ratio remains controversial in academia, but clearly we consume almost no omega-3 fat and massive excesses of omega-6 fats (more on this in the next chapter). Our diets have dramatically changed in the past century. We now consume almost no omega-3 fats while ingesting several grams of omega-6 fat daily.

Omega-3 fats are those involved in stopping inflammation; dampening down the immune response; calming our brains' reactions to excitatory input; keeping our blood appropriately thinned so we won't inappropriately clot in our brains (stroke), hearts (heart attack), legs (deep vein thrombosis), or lungs (pulmonary embolism); reducing the risk of dementia; improving vision; and slowing the development of macular degeneration. The list isn't yet completely defined, because it keeps growing each year.

Because our bodies can't make omega-3 fats, we need to consume them regularly to keep the inflammation in our bodies in check, ensure our immune systems are strong, keep our brains and nervous systems running smoothly, and prevent our blood from clotting when it shouldn't. Failure to do so could lead to any or all of these maladies, which would dramatically affect our quality of life. Often the outcome is premature death. Isn't it surprising that most people don't know about the importance of omega-3 fats in their diets?

Where are omega-3 fats found in our food chain? Prior to 1962, we consumed unpasteurized whole milk produced from grass-fed cows. This milk was rich in omega-3 fats. In 1962, the federal government mandated the pasteurization of milk. As a result, most farmers couldn't afford to establish dairy plants to pasteurize their milk. Most of the twenty million dairy farms went out of business due to this mandate. Many cows were moved to corporate dairy farms on massive feedlots. Cows that had once grazed on grass pastures (rich in omega-3 fat) were now fed corn silage and soybean meal (both are rich in omega-6 fats). Over time the levels of omega-3 fats found in meats and dairy products declined, and the omega-6 fat content increased.

Additionally, the pasteurization and homogenization processes destroy much omega-3 fat found in milk. Heat (pasteurization and now ultra-pasteurization) damaged or destroyed omega-3 fat. This caused more deficiency of this essential fat. When milk was pasteurized, it also destroyed many of the vitamins as well. Most Americans at the time supplemented their diet with cod liver oil to get enough vitamins A and D, since they didn't get adequate amounts of these vitamins if they didn't consume unpasteurized milk. With the urbanization of the United States, many people living in cities no longer had access to fresh milk; hence, the vitamin deficiencies. The Food and Drug Administration mandated the addition of these two important vitamins (A and D) to pasteurized milk, and cod liver oil consumption disappeared. Cod liver oil is rich in vitamins A and D, and it was also a significant source of omega-3 fat in our diets. Now that source is lost as well. So while we kept our vitamins A and D through supplementation, we lost a major source of omega-3 fats.

The homogenization process was implemented at the same time that milk was subjected to pasteurization. The milk is treated with intense pressure, which breaks up the butterfat. This damages butterfat and leads to decreased absorption of vitamins A and D. The cream no longer separates from the milk, and we lose the nutritional benefit of fat-soluble vitamin absorption seen with vitamins A and D. Our eyesight and bones have paid the price. I will explain more on saturated fat in another chapter.

A fascinating phenomenon has been discovered in the Greenland

Eskimos. They don't suffer from eye or bone disease. They aren't vitamin D deficient in spite of the lack of sunshine in this Arctic region of the world (sunshine enhances vitamin D production and absorption). They live on a diet rich in vitamin D and omega-3 fats. Consequently, even without adequate sun exposure for vitamin D activation, they have enough omega-3 fat to perform the same function. Omega-3 fats protect our eyes from macular degeneration and prevent osteoporosis and arthritis through anti-inflammatory mechanisms. Additionally, saturated fats enhance the absorption of vitamins A and D. The Arctic diet is rich in saturated fats as well as the omega-3 fish oils. Consequently, they are devoid of diseases we suffer from; eye and bone diseases are just two examples. They also are spared the ravages of cancer and heart disease as long as they continue living on their native diet.

Any food that is dark green or anything that consumes these dark-green vegetables as a mainstay of its diet contains omega-3 fats. In the ocean, algae and phytoplankton trap carbon dioxide during their bloom in the summertime with a process known as photosynthesis. The green of plants (chlorophyll) enables through photosynthesis the production of energy for the plant. Algae produce an abundance of omega-3 fat. Krill (a tiny shrimp) consume this fat in algae, and whales and feeder fish (herring, smelt, and mackerel) then consume them. Salmon eat the feeder fish, and we eat salmon and other fish in this food chain. Crabs, lobsters, clams, oysters, and the like consume the degradation of plant and animal life in the sea; this process ensures the delivery of other sea life we also enjoy in our culinary pleasures, all the while supplying us with omega-3 fats.

Carbon dioxide is the key ingredient to produce abundant sea life, and it all focuses around omega-3 fat production. Sea life is a prime source of omega-3 fat, and algae are the most abundant source on the planet. An abundance of this gas, produced by the degradation of plant and animal life, forest fires, volcanic action, and the like, is trapped by algae during photosynthesis and is the primary source of omega-3 production on the planet. With all the talk of global warming from excess carbon dioxide production and efforts to reduce levels of this gas, doesn't it strike you as odd that carbon dioxide is essential for healthy plant life? And healthy green plant life is essential to human health. Without carbon dioxide production, we would all perish. It isn't some evil gas we need to be punished for producing; it's the vital substance that allows all plant and animal life on the planet to thrive without significant disease. Without carbon dioxide, no carbon-based life forms, including us, could exist.

On land the same trapping of carbon dioxide occurs in plants to produce omega-3 fat, but different plants produce more omega-3 fat than others. Grains such as flax and chia are very rich in this essential fat. Corn, oats, and wheat have little or no omega-3 fat, while soybeans contain a mixture of both omega-3 and omega-6 fats. Dark-green vegetables and grasses also contain omega-3 fats. When insects, poultry, farm animals, and humans consume omega-3-rich plant foods, we all derive benefits from this anti-inflammatory oil. If a cow eats grasses and grains rich in omega-3 fats, we get omega-3 fats in our diets from its meat or milk products. If chickens eat bugs, greens, and grains rich in the same fat, we get omega-3 fat from eating their eggs or meat. If a pig eats greens from the garden, its meat is rich in omega-3 fat. You start to get the picture; we are what we eat. And we are also what farm animals, fowl, or fish eat.

Just how important is omega-3 fat to the diets of those who consume them? When we started producing farm-raised salmon, we quickly learned that if we tried to feed them food that was low in omega-3 fat, they died. Their diet must include food sources rich in omega-3 fat for them to survive on the fish farm. As I pointed out, wild salmon live on a diet rich in omega-3 fat. Studies now show that farm-raised salmon have nearly the same content of omega-3 fat in their bodies as wild salmon. If they don't consume an omega-3-rich diet, they just die, and we are without the farm-raised fish crop. So you purists can rest assured that farm-raised salmon are nearly as healthy for you as wild salmon, because fish farmers have learned that we cannot circumvent nature in this situation, as we've done with cows, chickens, and pigs.

Interestingly, cattle farmers have also seen the deterioration of the health of their animals when they are fed diets rich in omega-6 fats but deficient in omega-3 fats. Unfortunately, the difference isn't as stark as seen with the salmon farmers. Most cattle farmers still house their cattle on feedlots and feed them diets rich in corn and soybeans. This cheaper diet is rich in omega-6 fat instead of the omega-3-rich diets. Rather than keeping animals and us healthy on a diet rich in omega-3 fats (grasses, flax meal), this dietary change has been one of the contributing factors to America's deteriorating health from inflammatory diseases, heart diseases, and cancer. A push by the Food and Drug Administration and Department of Agriculture to return to a diet supplemented in omega-3 foods would go a long way toward improving the health of farm animals and producing farm foods that would be much healthier for all of us.

In the early 1960s, the Western diet underwent a series of changes that, for many people, destroyed our natural immunity and our ability to maintain a strong nervous system; many medical problems began to dominate the human condition. One of those changes was the significant loss of omega-3 fats from our diets. It took me a decade of homework in the National Library of Medicine to piece the story together. One of the most important pieces of that very complicated puzzle was the significant effects our bodies suffer when we don't consume enough omega-3 fats in our diets. It's important for us to understand that when we don't consume enough omega-3 fat, our bodies suffer numerous consequences. Those costs include autism in our children, depression surrounding pregnancy, bipolar disease in children and adults alike, sudden death from heart disease, immune dysfunction, and dementia, to name a few.

I've continued to monitor the medical literature, and evidence continues to mount, demonstrating the vital importance of including this fat regularly in our diets. Occasionally, studies are published showing that omega-3 fats don't cure a specific chronic disease. But in reality chronic diseases have multifactorial issues. An essential component of nutritional health or even a specific disease may be reversed by correcting an omega-3 fat deficiency. But that isn't always the case with multifactorial diseases, so tying their cure to omega-3 fats alone is why they fail.

One such study was published about the inability to cure Crohn's disease with omega-3 oil. Crohn's disease is a chronic inflammatory disease influenced by genetic factors, our immunologic state, and our diets. Inflammation can develop anywhere in the digestive tract, skin, joints, or liver. Treating such a complicated disease with a diet supplemented with omega-3 fat will certainly try to reduce inflammation, but to ignore other detrimental dietary habits that increase inflammation may defeat the purpose. The referenced study didn't use an adequate dose of omega-3 oil to meet normal requirements to keep our bodies healthy, and it didn't reduce omega-6 fats or trans fats (both known to worsen disease activity in Crohn's disease). This would be like treating a bladder infection with something ineffective against infections, such as iron therapy. Iron is needed to prevent anemia, but it doesn't prevent or treat infection. Additionally, if you treat a cancer with only a single course of chemotherapy when it may require eight courses of several chemical agents to eradicate the malady, don't ignore the fact that the treatment would have worked if implemented properly.

Omega-3 fat is the parent molecule the body uses to strengthen our immune system and reduce inflammation, but it isn't a drug that treats specific diseases. The study suggests to me that the researchers were ignorant about the importance of an essential oil, which is a building block for strengthening the anti-inflammatory arm of the immune system and maintaining an intact nervous system. Regardless, it was a waste of valuable research money spent trying to treat a genetically derived disease with an essential fat, which reduces inflammation seen in Crohn's disease but doesn't account for the dietary intake of pro-inflammatory fats, which exacerbate flares of the disease.

Studies like these, found in the medical literature, do nothing but cloud the science. They do nothing to improve our health, let alone advance our understanding of the science of medicine. I would never think of treating a disease with a multivitamin unless the disease was due to a specific deficiency. Treating scurvy with vitamin C would be appropriate, because scurvy is a disease resulting from no vitamin C in our diets. The deficiency would kill us in about six weeks. Vitamin C therapy reverses scurvy. Likewise, omega-3 oil will prevent and, in some cases, reverse specific diseases related to its deficiency. Fish oil can both prevent and treat postpartum depression. Fish oil can also treat and prevent osteoporosis; it can also prevent and treat macular degeneration. Many other examples can be found in the medical literature.

Crohn's disease is a genetic disease that can be made worse with omega-3 fat deficiency, but adding omega-3 fat to our diets doesn't correct the genetic defects and may not even prevent flares in the disease from occurring if other triggers, such as excess consumption of trans fats or omega-6 oil, block the beneficial effects of omega-3 fat. Additionally, if chronic omega-3 deficiency has damaged our immune system, this may not necessarily be repaired with omega-3 supplementation. More research needs to be done in this area so we can give our patients better advice concerning dietary management of inflammatory diseases, such as Crohn's disease, rheumatoid arthritis, psoriasis, and the like.

As I pointed out in the previous chapter, trans fats block the metabolic function of omega-3 fat. If you're trying to improve your health by getting an adequate portion of omega-3 fat in your diet while continuing to consume trans fat, you're losing ground to the harmful effects of trans fats. Additionally, if we overwhelm our metabolism with excess omega-6 fat, the metabolism of omega-3 fat cannot compete to keep our health strong. A common enzyme processes omega-3 and omega-6 fat through the liver. If omega-3 fat gets there first, it's preferentially processed. Ingesting omega-6 before omega-3 fat or in excess in your meal (deep-fried fish and chips, for example), this suppresses omega-3 metabolism. In turn, you've lost any benefit you may have derived from the omega-3 fat in the fish while delighting in your omega-6 deep-fried meal.

It's very important to understand that some medical conditions can be prevented or treated with omega-3 fats. I want to explore this a bit further with you. An example is post-partum depression. Studies reveal that this type of depression is due to a deficiency of this fat. Omega-3 fat is a major component of our brains. When a woman is pregnant and her diet is deficient of this essential fat, omega-3 fat is mobilized from her brain and passed to the fetus. After delivery, the mother's milk is enriched by the omega-3 fat stored in her body and passed to the baby. If the mom is consuming omega-3 fats in her diet, there's no problem. But if she is deficient, then the omega-3 fat is taken from her brain, transferred to the breast milk, and sent on to the baby. The problem is that when our brains are depleted of omega-3 fat, we see several short-term and long-term effects: depression, bipolar disorders, autism, neuropathy, and dementia. If they are caught early enough, some conditions are reversible. Likewise, if enough damage has occurred to our nervous system, there is permanent loss in some aspects of our nervous system function.

The same holds true for inflammatory conditions that occur because we're omega-3 fat deficient. One of the best examples of this, which I have personally seen and is well published, is the effects of psoriasis. This inflammatory skin and joint condition can be remedied in some people with the addition of omega-3 oil in an otherwise-deficient diet. Likewise, if the disease process has been present in an uncontrolled state for too long, skin and joint destruction may be too advanced to be corrected. Finally, omega-6 fats and trans fats are inflammatory and must be reduced to maximize the benefits of omega-3 fat in this situation as well.

There has been an explosion of inflammatory diseases in the past sixty years since we became deficient in omega-3 fat intake in the 1960s. While this is a huge component of this upsurge of these diseases, there are other components that contribute to this problem as well. These include the excess consumption of omega-6 and trans fats. We need to simultaneously supplement our diets with omega-3 fats while ridding it of trans fats and dramatically reducing omega-6 intake. It's the implementation of this triad that produces the most effective results to improve the anti-inflammatory response, at the same time decreasing the pro-inflammatory response of our diets to our immune system.

Many medications have been developed in the past fifty years to treat inflammatory diseases, heart disease, and bone thinning. But physicians, for the most part, don't ensure that their patients are consuming an adequate amount of omega-3 fats in their diets. The result is that more and more people require more medications to treat those inflammatory diseases, heart disease, and bone thinning, while these same individuals are deficient in the one nutrient in their diet that is required to prevent or naturally reduce the disease process in the first place. One of the best examples of this is heart disease. Numerous prospective studies show that adding fish, fish oil, or flax oil to people who suffer from heart disease, are "at risk" of heart disease, or are omega-3 fat deficient benefit from omega-3 supplementation. Studies consistently demonstrate a reduction of 40 to 50 percent in heart disease in long-term follow-up.

Consensus of the American Heart Association, federal government agencies, and numerous international scientific organizations and academic nutritional experts now all acknowledge that omega-3 fat intake on a regular basis reduces heart attacks and sudden death from heart disease. In 1996 the American Heart Association included guidelines on their website that promoted the consumption of fish for "at risk" individuals. At the same time, they and others emphasized that saturated fats and cholesterol were the prime cause of heart disease. This conclusion is confusing, to say the least, especially in light of the fact that we learned from the Food and Drug Administration in February 2015 that we no longer need to concern ourselves with the cholesterol content in our food.

Treatment of heart disease has focused on lowering cholesterol with statin therapy. These statin medications (Lipitor, Pravachol, Zocor, Mevacor, and so forth) reduces LDL cholesterol, and this effect was thought to be the primary reason there is a therapeutic benefit. While the statin medications lower cholesterol, they also have a thinning effect on blood and reduce inflammation. These are the same benefits derived from the natural omega-3 fats found in fish, flax, and greens without the potentially dangerous side effects reported with statin therapy. Some of the most dangerous toxicities reported with statin use include cancer (breast and prostate), dementia, transient global amnesia, and muscle damage. Why wouldn't someone want to have the same results without the toxic side effects?

Aspirin has also been used to prevent heart attacks, and this medication thins the blood to reduce the number of blood clots in the heart's arteries, but it also needs to be taken indefinitely like statins. Like other medications, aspirin carries risks from continued use, and these include peptic ulcer disease, bleeding, kidney damage, and death.

Omega-3 fat deficiency has been recognized only in the past few decades, while loss of this essential fat from our diets occurred in epidemic proportions in the sixties. As the science of fat physiology has grown, so also has the understanding of the importance of omega-3 fat. The primary, parent omega-3 fat is alpha-linolenic acid (ALA). This oil is found in dark-green plants, chia, flax, soybeans, and nuts but not much in animals or fish. Our livers convert the ALA we consume from these food sources to docosahexaenoic acid (DHA) and eicosapentaenoic acid

(EPA). Then it is stored in the membranes of our cells until needed to maintain our health.

The same conversion of ALA to DHA and EPA occurs when fish, animals, and birds consume ALA in their diets. If we then eat those food sources, we ingest DHA and EPA. Plants don't make the conversion of ALA to EPA and DHA. They produce, store and then consume the ALA as an energy source for cell replication and growth. When we eat plants, our livers convert the ALA to EPA and DHA as long as we consume appropriate vitamins and have a healthy liver.

The source of omega-3 fat in our diets is clearly a food choice. A vegetarian can get adequate omega-3s from plant sources so long as he or she has a healthy liver. Meat eaters can get the same from omega-3-rich animal, bird, or fish sources. Much is written about which omega-3 fat is best for us. Some argue that we need DHA and EPA, but vegans survive without eating animals, birds, or fish that are rich in these fats. They consume ALA from only plant sources. I advise patients to try to mix it up if possible from various food sources and supplements, as each of us tolerates omega-3 fats from various food sources in varying degrees. Some people thrive on fish oil, while others burp it excessively. Others complain that they smell like fish when they consume it. Flax oil gives some individuals diarrhea. Either way, all these are excellent sources of omega-3 fats.

If we're deficient in DHA, we'll suffer from neurological problems. Likewise, if we're deficient in EPA, we'll have problems combating inflammation in its many forms. If our livers function appropriately and we have no genetic disorders that prevent the conversion of ALA to DHA and EPA, our bodies will make the necessary conversions of ALA to these latter oils, as the body requires. Why this is important is that some people are unable to tolerate or are allergic to fish oil (ALA and DHA), so they must get their omega-3 source from plant-based sources, such as flax, chia, nuts, or eggs and animal products from omega-3-fortified sources. Flax and chia primarily contain ALA, while eggs and animals fortified with ALA sources primarily contain DHA and EPA. Some grains such as quinoa contain omega-3 fat, but they also contain ten times the amount of omega-6 fat.

The importance of incorporating omega-3 fats into our diets in the proper balance with omega-6 fats cannot be understated. We should try to consume some of this fat at each meal and preferably at the beginning of the meal, as it competes in the liver with trans fat and omega-6 fat through the same metabolic pathway. If it gets to the liver first, it will be preferentially metabolized. If it is consumed after either of these other fats, it loses out. All you have to do is consume the omega-3 before the omega-6 fat to give the omega-3 fat an advantage in your body's metabolic and immune activities. Additionally, excess omega-6 or trans fat ingestion can overwhelm omega-3 fat processing in the liver which deprives us of the benefits of consuming the omega-3 fatty acids.

At least one patient questions me nearly every day about how much omega-3 fat he or she should take. If you go to the FDA website, omega-3 fatty acids aren't given a recommended daily allowance. I find this odd since every other known essential nutrient is listed with a guideline. Because of the way our food production has changed since the development of trans fats and the movement away from grass-fed to corn-fed animals, we consume too much omega-6 fat in our diets. Our bodies require a balance of these two oils for proper immune function, inflammation control, and neurological function; it's essential to dramatically lower omega-6 fatty acid intake to about one gram per day and consume at least two to four grams of omega-3 fatty acid per day to achieve this balance. We presently consume over forty grams of omega-6 oil per day and almost no omega-3 fat. (At least twenty to forty grams of omega-3 fat would be necessary to balance the effects of that much omega-6 fat.) Several studies document this in blood tests. Our bodies store these two oils in our cells. The American population currently reveals an omega-6/omega-3 ratio of 14-17/1. This ratio should be about 1-2/1. This is due to two facts: in our diets, we don't get enough omega-3 fat, and we get too much omega-6 fat.

Unfortunately, the food label isn't yet required to show the amount of omega-3 fat content from the foods we consume. There are foods available that do include the omega-3 content, such as eggs, but this is a means to advertise that fact so we might choose them over a different brand. If the label reveals the presence of omega-3, it gives you another choice in your diet where you can consume this essential oil without requiring additional supplementation. If the food label doesn't designate it, use the rule of thumb that fish is good, grass fed is good, and saturated fats like butter are good. Avoid processed food as much as possible. If you cannot afford the higher prices of omega-3-rich foods, buy some flaxseed, krill, or fish oil and take that before meals to ensure your body selects the omega-3 over the omega-6 oil. Finally, completely eliminate trans fats from your diet. These are found only in processed foods.

Pearls

- Omega-3 fats are essential to our health.
- Our bodies don't produce omega-3 fats, so we must consume them daily.
- Omega-3 fat deficiency leads to many diseases and premature death.
- The balance between omega-3 and omega-6 fats is vital.
- We need to learn how to supplement our diets with omega-3 fats.

CHAPTER 3

Reduce Omega-6 Fatty Acids

We occasionally stumble over the truth but most of us pick
ourselves up and hurry off as if nothing had happened.
Winston Churchill

So you and your child or grandchild finally arrives at the local
fishing hole, and you bring along worms as bait to attract the fish
to your hook. The only problem is that today the fish are biting only on
grasshoppers. You don't have any grasshoppers, so you keep fishing with
worms, hoping your luck might just land a fish or two. Likewise, when
you go to the grocery store today, nearly all processed food contains
some sort of omega-6 oil. You've been told that too much omega-6 oil
is bad for you, but perhaps if you just eat a little bit, it won't negatively
affect you. The only "bait" in your favorite processed foods is made with
soybean oil, cottonseed oil, sunflower oil, peanut oil, rapeseed (canola)
oil, safflower oil, or corn oil. What is the big deal anyway?

What all these oils have in common is that when they are used
in processed foods, they contain a very high content of omega-6 fat.
As you learned in the previous chapter, omega-6 fat (also known as
linoleic acid) is an essential fat. This fat is the parent oil converted to
arachidonic acid, which is then converted to inflammatory compounds

necessary to fight infection, wounds, burns, and the like. The problem comes when we consume too much of this oil on a daily basis. That is exactly what has happened in the American diet over the past sixty years. We now ingest nearly forty grams of these oils per day, and they are wreaking havoc on our immune system, joints, blood vessels, brain and nervous system, intestinal tract, and skin. You guessed it; our entire body is inflamed because of this excess omega-6 fat.

In my first book, *42 Days to a New Life*, I outlined nearly all the diseases that develop because of excess daily omega-6 fat consumption. What's important to realize is that we need to learn to read the food label to determine what "bait" we're taking home from the grocery store, whether our food has high omega-6 content. The first thing to do is find out which oil is being used in the food item you're interested in buying. All processed vegetable oil is primarily omega-6 fat. Heating such an oil damages or destroys most of the omega-3 fatty acids that may have been present in it.

An excellent example of this is processed foods containing soybean oil. Unprocessed soybean oil contains both omega-3 and omega-6 fat. Processing the soybean oil destroys most, if not all, of the omega-3 portion and leaves the processed food with the omega-6 fat. Heat and light destroy omega-3 fats, so they don't preserve food well for a prolonged life on the grocery store shelf. Food items that contain omega-3 fats need to be consumed within days to just a few weeks after processing, or they will become rancid, and the food will taste bad. Think about a fresh fish at the market. It quickly becomes rancid and unfit for consumption, as the smell of a "bad" fish reminds us all too well.

Omega-6 fat isn't affected by heat or light in the same manner as omega-3 fatty acids. Consequently, that bag of potato chips, tortillas, cookies, crackers, cakes, breads, and so forth will remain edible for a much longer duration when produced with omega-6 oil. And as we all know, you can't eat just one "serving size," as listed on the food label.

This takes me to the next point concerning the food label. We need to see how much omega-6 fat we are consuming when we dive into that bag of potato chips. Typically, we might consume three or four "servings," and by doing so, we may ingest several grams of omega-6 fat in just a few minutes. One serving of potato chips (thirteen to seventeen chips) contains approximately one gram of omega-6 fat. That is all your body needs to remain healthy for the entire day. And while you're sitting in front of the television, consumed by your favorite movie, football game, and so forth, have you ever counted out fifteen chips?

Now compound that diet with our consumption of fried foods found in the fast-food industry (remember; only the omega-6 fats and trans fats survive the deep-frying process). Breads and pastries are now being baked with vegetable oils, many salad dressings and other condiments are prepared with omega-6 oils, and most snack foods are produced with these same oils. The list goes on, and by the end of the day we've easily consumed thirty to forty grams of omega-6 fat. As a side note, before we switched to trans fats and vegetable oils, processed and fast foods were cooked in farm fats, palm oil and coconut oil. When I performed a quick Google search, I found that the average American frequents fast-food restaurants 2.6 times per week, and he or she dines out an average of four to five times per week. That doesn't include home delivery of pizza or other processed foods. About three billion pizzas are sold annually in America. If you personalize these numbers, you can quickly see that your diet is overwhelmed with omega-6 fats.

Another very important problem with consuming omega-6 fat-laden foods from fast-food restaurants is that these oils undergo a dangerous transformation into toxic compounds when heated to high temperatures in a deep fryer. When you consume french fries or deep-fried fish, you eat compounds known as MCPDs (monochloropropane diol and glycodiol esters). MCPDs have been discovered to cause cancer and kidney disease. Another compound produced with the heating of omega-6 oils is HNE (4-hydroxynonenol). The importance of this compound in causing toxicity to humans has been become clear since the 1990s. Data now show that HNE consumption causes neurodegenerative diseases such as Parkinson's disease, increased cholesterol, increased inflammation, and body protein loss.

Data are now emerging that compounds such as MCPDs and HNE may place fast-food workers at increased risk of developing lung cancer from chronic exposure to aerosolized omega-6 fats coming out of the deep-fat fryers. It will be interesting to follow the literature in the future as more and more toxic compounds are being discovered and investigated from the heating of omega-6 oils. In the meantime, I recommend that you stop consuming deep-fried foods and avoid exposing yourself to a workplace that deep fries or excessively heats foods in these oils.

Our bodies may be able to handle this excess of omega-6 fat on occasion, but when we consume this much inflammatory oil on a daily basis, as is the case for many Americans, it begins to take a heavy toll on our health. We are seeing an explosion of autoimmune disorders (autoimmune thyroiditis, systemic lupus, mixed connective tissue disease, rheumatoid arthritis, scleroderma, Sjögren's disease, and so forth), inflammatory skin diseases (psoriasis, acne, eczema, and so forth), joint problems (osteoarthritis, osteoporosis, joint failure, and so forth), intestinal problems (esophageal reflux, celiac disease, Crohn's disease, ulcerative colitis, microscopic colitis, and so forth), blood vessel disease (heart disease, stroke, peripheral vascular disease, and so forth), and brain and nerve problems (ADD, ADHD, autism, depression, bipolar disease, Parkinson's disease, dementias, and so forth). The list of inflammatory diseases is now center stage in the health care arena. While many of these disorders have multifactorial risk factors in the expression of their disease, the medical literature has overwhelmingly documented a direct link between these diseases and excess consumption of omega-6 oil.

As a gastroenterologist, I monitor the medical literature pertinent to my specialty. When I investigated this topic for my first book, I was astonished to learn that the daily excess omega-6 and trans fats found in our diets exacerbated all the inflammatory diseases I'd researched. Compound this by the deficiency of omega-3 fatty acids in our diets, which tries to reduce inflammation in our bodies and creates the perfect storm. None of this information is revealed in biochemistry, physiology, pathology, or internal medicine textbooks. All my resources were found squirreled away in the National Library of Medicine, dying a silent inflammatory death.

While I could overwhelm you with data, I have vowed not to do so with this book. Rather, my goal is to give you a big-picture overview, and when I need to prove a point, I'll try to include an example or two. One such example is a large cohort of people who've been prospectively followed in Europe (about two hundred fifty thousand). It has been determined that those who consume fast food regularly are seeing a doubling of ulcerative colitis annually in their population compared to those who don't eat fast food. Even where trans fat has been eliminated in the fast-food industry (McDonald's stopped using trans fats several years ago), the fries, deep-fried chicken or fish, and other fried foods are all prepared in omega-6-rich oils. You will often consume several grams of this inflammatory oil in a single meal. Repeating this behavior several times per week eventually inflames our bodies in a multitude of ways. If this process persists long enough, we end up suffering irreversible consequences of this inflammation.

A patient of mine suffers from Crohn's disease. He could cause his disease to flare by consuming french-fried potatoes. While he suffers from a genetically based inflammatory disorder of his intestinal tract, he has learned that he can keep it under much better control by avoiding this and other inflammatory foods.

In addition to the inflammatory issues related to omega-6 oils, someone recently stated that by consuming deep-fried foods that have been cooked in omega-6 vegetable oils, we ingest oxidized fatty acids produced from the oil being heated to high temperatures. These oxidized fats generate free radicals (unstable and highly reactive molecules that can damage cells) in our bodies. Data now show that these can lead to cancer. Antioxidants, those occurring naturally in our bodies and those consumed in foods and beverages, try to protect us from getting cancer. But if you look at the explosion of breast, colon, skin, and prostate cancer and lymphomas in the past fifty years, you'll notice that we clearly haven't been protected from these diseases. It will be interesting to see how the Food and Drug Administration, agribusiness, and the academic nutrition community deal with this information in the next few years, as more people begin reducing their intake of these fried-oil food products.

I need to interject an important thought at this point about saturated fats as they relate to omega-6 fats. I have a separate chapter about saturated fats, but some explanation is warranted here. Our livers convert saturated fats to oleic acid (olive oil) derivatives. Oleic acid (also called omega-9 fatty acid) is the primary oil found in olive oil, and many organizations and the federal government have deemed it "heart healthy." This would suggest an obvious contradiction. It took me some time to unravel this mystery, and I had to venture into the veterinary medicine and agriculture literature to sort out the conundrum. It comes down to the adage that "you are what you eat" when it comes to fats. If a grass-fed cow is changed to corn silage and soybean meal (both rich in omega-6 fat), the cow's meat composition transforms from omega-3-rich fat (if the animal was grass fed) to omega-6-rich meat. Both animals contain the same saturated fat content, but one animal's meat is anti-inflammatory (omega-3, grass fed), while the other inflames (omega-6, corn and soybean fed) our bodies. Likewise, if chickens eat bugs (rich in omega-3 fat), flax meal, or other sources of omega-3 fat, their meat and eggs will be anti-inflammatory, and if they are fed cornmeal, their food products will be inflammatory.

You start to see why it has taken so long to sort out the confusion about saturated fats. Modern scientific data show that saturated fats consumed from palm oil, coconut oil, and the like aren't the problem with fat consumption in the American diet. It's the inappropriately excessive consumption of omega-6 fats and trans fats along with an omega-3 fat deficiency. A three-and-a half-ounce piece of chinook (king) salmon and the same-sized piece of New York strip steak have the same saturated fat content of about three grams. Yet we are told that salmon is our friend, while the beefsteak is our enemy. An entire food and health care industry is built on this omega-fat imbalance, saturated-fat confusion, and toxic manufactured trans fat consumption. Now it's difficult for us to figure out how to get the problem resolved.

So what have we learned so far? We've discovered that trans fats are hydrogenated vegetable oils that seriously damage our health and must be eliminated. Next, we learned that omega-3 fat is an essential oil necessary for reducing inflammation and preserving nerve function. We once consumed a diet rich in this fat, but that all changed in the 1960s. We're now an omega-3-fat-deficient nation and need to find supplemental ways to negate that deficit. Finally, we've dramatically increased our omega-6 fat intake, and this has led to an explosion of inflammatory diseases, heart problems, and cancers. We must correct all these problems if we are to live healthier lives.

First is to eliminate all trans fats from our diets. Second, we must increase omega-3 fat intake. Finally, we need to dramatically reduce omega-6 fat consumption. We should avoid deep-fat-fried foods, but this can create a challenge when dining out. We need to train ourselves to make better choices in this regard. We can choose grilled foods, salads dressed with vinegars and olive oil, soups, and entrees that are baked rather than fried. When we cook at home, we need to learn to bake and fry with butter, coconut oil, palm oil, and olive oil. Lastly, we need to learn to read the ingredient section of the food label to ensure we're not consuming hydrogenated or partially hydrogenated vegetable oils (trans fats).

We need to move away from processed foods made with corn, cottonseed, safflower, canola, peanut, and soybean oil. These oils are rich in omega-6 fat. If enough consumers change their eating habits, we'll see a change in the processed foods industry. This change has already begun to occur in the gluten-free food choices. Develop the habit of taking omega-3 supplements (fish, flax, or krill) twice daily at the beginning of the meal with a daily multivitamin if you don't have access to omega-3-rich foods. When shopping, look for grass-fed beef, omega-3-enriched eggs, fresh fish, and the like when your budget allows. Most importantly, make this a lifestyle change, not a fad diet.

Pearls

- Omega-6 fats are essential for our health.
- We consume about forty times more than we need.
- Excess omega-6 fat intake leads to inflammatory diseases, cancer, heart disease, and premature death.
- We need to limit our omega-6 fat (vegetable oils) intake to one to two grams per day.

CHAPTER 4

Reduce Fructose Consumption

Facts are stubborn things; and whatever may be our
wishes, our inclinations, or the dictates of our passions,
they cannot alter the state of facts and evidence.
John Adams

When my grandmother was growing up in the rural North Idaho panhandle, she would mount her horse and ride that mare to school several miles from her farm every day. She was one of several children in a family that didn't have electricity, a refrigerator, a freezer, processed foods, jet planes bringing fresh kiwi fruit from New Zealand, or nitrogen warehouses storing fresh fruit so it could be consumed year round. She related to me that her family would can some foodstuffs, since most people couldn't afford to buy canned foods from grocery stores. The family had a barnyard full of chickens, a milk cow, horses for transportation, and a large garden and orchard. Life was simple and hard, but no one went without, and she lived to be ninety-six years old. Her only health problem until she died was mild high blood pressure in old age.

Why do I tell you this story? It's because as a child she grew up without much in the way of daily excess fructose consumption. It was a way of life for her and millions of other Americans. Contrast that time to today; our daily fructose consumption comes from fruit, juices, honey, sugar, and high-fructose-corn-syrup-containing beverages, condiments, pastries, breads, cookies, candies, and the like. Worse, the US Department of Agriculture, the Food and Drug Administration, and other civilian and government organizations advise us to consume a diet laden with this sugar. The food pyramid and now the MyPlate (the most recent dietary guideline published by the United States Department of Agriculture in 2010) guidelines advise us to consume more fructose than our bodies can handle, and this practice is having harmful effects on our health.

Fructose, also known as fruit sugar, is found in most fruits. A modern hybridized apple contains enough fructose to overwhelm one's metabolism for over twenty-four hours. You see, the liver metabolizes fructose and converts it to blood glucose when we consume very small quantities. Our livers can handle about ten to fifteen grams of fructose per day and keep up with this biochemical conversion process. Once we exceed that quantity on a daily basis, it takes about six days to two weeks to turn on an alternative metabolic pathway that converts the fructose into triglycerides (fat). Once this pathway is turned on, the liver now preferentially converts all fructose we consume into this fat.

An apple of the size I grew up eating on our family farm contained less than ten grams of fructose. It was crisp and tart with low sugar content. A modern apple contains more than double that amount. Now compound that information with the advice to eat several servings of fruit per day (a banana has eight grams; an orange, seven grams; a pear, twelve grams; a slice of watermelon, twelve grams; and so forth), and you can easily exceed the amount your liver can handle. By following the MyPlate nutritional guidelines of fructose intake, adding several servings of fruit per day, and consuming other foods laden with fructose, you will soon hit the national average of about eighty grams per day. And that's by avoiding soda pop. If you throw in an additional twenty-ounce soda pop, you just shot over one hundred grams for the day.

The next time you're at a large shopping mall, look to see how many fruit smoothie stands are present with a line of young people waiting to consume nature's sugar. A typical medium-sized fruit smoothie will contain forty grams of fructose. Fructose consumption in America was about ten grams per person per day in 1960. We now consume more than eight times that much per day.

Fructose is a unique sugar when it comes to human history on our planet. First, the largest ecosystem on earth, the ocean, doesn't contain any appreciable fructose. Second, while fruit was found in isolated pockets on earth, it was found in very low content. When President Thomas Jefferson commissioned Meriwether Lewis to carry out the Lewis and Clark expedition in 1804, part of his mission was to document the plant life of the North American continent. The only fruits found in America were crab apples, wild strawberries, wild blackberries, and huckleberries. As you know, these fruits are very tart and don't contain much fructose. They are also very small compared to the modern hybridized varieties we find at the supermarket. I'm sure you've seen some strawberries that are nearly as big as a tangerine. Those were never part of nature.

The next point to remember is that table sugar wasn't part of the human diet until the last fifteen hundred years. This sugar is 50 percent fructose and was first crystalized from sugar cane around AD 350 in India. Christopher Columbus brought it to North America over one thousand years later. Sugar is now the largest crop on the planet, the United Nations reported in 2010. The early centuries after cane sugar was produced as a crop led to the production of alcohol, when it is fermented and then distilled. This is where rum comes from. By the time we learned how to ferment table sugar, we had already mastered fermentation of other fruits and vegetables into alcohol. Grapes were converted into wine; apples became hard cider; grains produced beer and ale. When we mastered the art of distillation, wine was turned into brandy, potatoes became vodka, and grains and corn became whiskeys.

Table sugar became a sweetener for foods and beverages only in the last few hundred years. In 1700 sugar consumption per capita in England was only four pounds per year; that number rose to 120 pounds per year by 1980. Little data is available on consumption of sugar until the twentieth century in America, but we now consume an average of 150 to 180 pounds of sugar per person each year.

This leads me to the next point, the laboratory production of fructose. This process was mastered in the 1960s, and by the end of the 1970s, mass production of fructose was in full swing in the United States. We've come to know this commodity at the grocery store as high-fructose corn syrup. Sugar is extracted from corn and then converted into fructose in the laboratory. It is then mixed with glucose (the same sugar that circulates in our veins) in appropriate concentrations to make high-fructose corn syrup. With the addition of this form of sugar into our Western diet, combined refined sugar and high-fructose-corn-syrup-derived sugar consumption rose to 150 pounds per person per year in 2000. That number has recently declined to about 130 to 135 pounds per person annually from its peak consumption of 180 pounds in 2009.

While we were increasing our intake of table sugar and high-fructose corn syrup, we also began to consume larger quantities of fruit, fruit juice. and honey (one of the richest sources of fructose). An interesting side note about honey is that the average American consumes about 1.4 pounds of this fructose-laden substance annually. That equals about eleven hundred grams of honey per year or about three grams per day. Honey contains sixteen times the amount of fructose in an apple by weight and is the richest source of fructose in our diets.

Rapid air transportation of fruits from exotic locations, nitrogen warehouses that can store fruit for extended periods of time before being consumed, and apiaries now found all over the planet have led to rapid increases in fructose intake. We now consume these fructose-rich foods and beverages year round. Before these technological changes, fructose intake was dictated by when fruit ripened and what could be obtained locally. Now an increased consumption of fructose from all sources far exceeds the digestive capacity of the intestines and liver.

Thousands of patients have asked me over the past three decades why excess fruit is unhealthy. Fruit is part of nature; it's rich in vitamins and minerals and serves as a great fiber source. I have to explain to them that fruit is "nature's candy," which was designed to be consumed in only small quantities, in small concentrations (as was found in nature before hybridization and genetic modification techniques were developed), and only in their season. We've somehow convinced ourselves that nature's candy is good for us. If I were to tell you to eat five bars of Snickers per day or a pound of M&M's daily, you would think I was off my rocker. Yet when we are told to consume the same amount or more of fructose from "nature's candy," we've tricked ourselves into believing this is healthy. My next chapter explains the metabolic disaster that is now an epidemic in America, and this relentless, excess daily fructose intake has primarily caused it. As I've also learned, there's more to this story as it relates to grains. Wheat contains a different kind of sugar called amylopectin that worsens the metabolic effects of excess fructose.

Fructose also wreaks havoc inside the intestines for many of us. I recently saw a woman who had been making trips to the local hospital emergency room for intense abdominal pains. Standard evaluations consistently revealed that nothing was wrong with her. She had blood tests, urine tests, electrocardiograms, CT scans, ultrasounds—you get the idea. I saw her husband, and in passing he asked me whether I could help. I noted in her medical record that just prior to her most recent visit to the hospital; she'd eaten an apple and pancakes with syrup. I gave her a copy of my book *Fructose Exposed*. She went home, read the book from cover to cover, and promptly changed her diet. She was consuming about eighty grams of fructose per day, and when she stopped this, her intestinal pains promptly stopped.

This is a story I hear regularly in my practice. There are several studies in the medical literature that describe fructose malabsorption and familial fructose intolerance. If you suffer from periodic abdominal pain for no apparent reason and have been evaluated with repeatedly negative answers, perhaps you also suffer from this problem. All it requires is for you to stop consuming fructose, and your symptoms will abate.

One difficulty of stopping fructose intake is that if we consume it daily in excess, it takes only a few weeks for us to become addicted to this sugar. Research studies reveal that fructose alters the natural blood flow in our brains, leading to a change in the hormone regulation of our appetites. This dysregulation causes us not to get the appropriate signals to our brains that should tell us we're not hungry. In turn, we continue to eat, even though we've consumed plenty of calories. This habit leads to overeating, obesity, and the multitude of metabolic changes that occur from this process. Additionally, as we will discuss in the next chapter, daily excess fructose intake leads to activation of the metabolic syndrome and its consequences.

One final point: many patients ask me why some people can consume more than ten to fifteen grams of fructose per day without any problems. Published data reveal that when we are involved in heavy physical exercise (soccer, mountain climbing, competitive bicycling, and so forth) or experiencing a growth spurt during the first two decades of our lives, our metabolisms can tolerate a bit more. But this is truly the exception for most of us, as witnessed by the fructose-induced epidemic of obesity, metabolic syndrome, and the plethora of associated diseases that are highly visible among our youth and adults alike.

Let's return to my grandmother at this juncture. She eventually had a refrigerator and freezer; she grew accustomed to the amenities of grocery store shopping; she was no longer required to figure out how to process and store food for the winter months. Yet she continued to live out of her garden and orchard. She also continued to consume farm food in the manner she had as a child. And for the ninety-six years she spent on this planet, she never adopted the modern consumption habits that prevail in America today. We certainly don't need to return to a time without electricity, refrigeration, and the like, but we definitely need to revert to the dietary habits of my grandmother's generation if we want to live healthier lives.

Pearls

- Our bodies can properly metabolize about ten to fifteen grams of fructose per day.
- The average daily consumption of fructose is presently about eighty grams per day.
- Fruit, fruit juice, honey, table sugar, and high-fructose corn syrup are the primary sources of fructose in our diets.
- Excessive daily consumption of fructose leads to metabolic syndrome, gastrointestinal distress, and sugar addiction.
- We need to limit our daily consumption of fructose to ten to fifteen grams per day.

CHAPTER 5

Metabolic Syndrome: Reverse It!

There does not exist a category of science to which one can give
the name applied science. There are science and the applications
of science, bound together as the fruit of the tree which bears it.

Louis Pasteur

At this juncture, one of those very important concepts all of us
need to understand, since it affects millions in America today,
is metabolic syndrome. If I were to tell you that a new infectious
disease was discovered that would slowly kill you without treatment or
vaccination, you would probably try to learn about that infection. In
today's instant knowledge availability, you would get on the Internet
and talk, text, or communicate through your favorite form of social
media to someone who knows more about the infection than you do.
You might learn to recognize the signs and symptoms of the infection.
Most likely, you would even warn your family and friends about
the potential perils of this "killer germ" before they fall prey to its
devastation. More importantly, if the disease affected seventy million
adults and millions more children and adolescents, it would clearly get
your attention. Imagine strolling through your local mall and realizing

that every fourth person you encountered was infected with this deadly disease.

Such is the case with metabolic syndrome, yet it's easily treatable. Like many infections, untreated metabolic syndrome will eventually kill us. Some die quickly from a heart attack or stroke; diabetes, cirrhosis of the liver, liver cancer, or liver failure ravages others. Others go into kidney failure and die or are kept alive by renal dialysis. Gout and its painful suffering afflict others. Diseases caused by its associated obesity consume other people's lives. Regardless of the sign or symptom of metabolic syndrome you or a loved one manifests, the outcome is the same: pain, suffering, and premature death without prevention or treatment.

Just what is metabolic syndrome? It's a clustering of medical problems that develop over a period of months to years due to daily, excess consumption of fructose. Those medical problems may include the following:

- Elevation of serum triglycerides
- Elevation of LDL cholesterol (considered "bad" cholesterol in medical literature)
- Reduction of HDL cholesterol (considered "good" cholesterol in medical literature)
- Increased waist circumference (called central obesity)
- High blood pressure
- Fatty liver
- Gout in predisposed individuals
- Type 2 diabetes

The first case of metabolic syndrome was described in 1947, and the disorder became a recognized medical condition in America by the 1980s. Today, nearly seventy million of us suffer from metabolic syndrome, and it now affects millions of children as well. How did we go from the first described patient with this malady to the epidemic occurring in the last half of the twentieth century? Many of our medical problems across America can be attributed to trans fats and excess omega-6 fat consumption, compounded by omega-3 fat deficiency. Daily excessive fructose intake has made matters even worse, bringing the dramatic rise of metabolic syndrome. The first three issues of fat imbalance lead to dysregulation of our immune system and markedly increase inflammation throughout our bodies. Excess daily intake of fructose alters our metabolisms in a way that creates a perfect storm for us to develop heart disease, stroke, diabetes, high blood pressure, kidney failure, fatty liver, cirrhosis, the consequences of obesity, and gout.

It was only in the last decade that the metabolic changes that occur when we consume too much daily fructose were beginning to unravel. The initial chemical changes occur in only six days to two weeks and require only twenty-five grams or less of daily fructose intake in most of us. We've all met the individual who can eat anything and get away with it, but the other 90 percent of us are vulnerable to this problem. What happens? The fructose from our apple, soda pop, honey in our cup of tea (it doesn't matter the source) is taken into the liver from the intestine, where it is converted to triglyceride (a form of fat that accumulates in our abdomen area and liver). While this occurs, it switches off production of HDL ("good") cholesterol and increases production of LDL and VLDL ("bad") cholesterol. These changes occur within two to six weeks of daily, excessive consumption of fructose. The waste product of this fructose-to-fat conversion is the production of uric acid.

Uric acid is the stuff that causes gout in the genetically predisposed person. A buildup of this waste product can occur in many of us without our suffering from the genetic form of gout. This occurs when we consume large quantities of fructose on a daily basis. Excessive uric acid affects the kidneys in a negative way. It causes the kidneys to retain salt, and this, in turn, leads to the retention of water, which leads to high blood pressure. Have you ever wondered why you lose five pounds when you initiate a strict diet to lose weight? When you stop consuming the excess fructose you consume daily, uric acid production precipitously drops. This allows the kidneys to release the salt in our urine, and with it goes our excess water. Studies in children who suffer from metabolic syndrome have demonstrated that they immediately drop their blood pressure by about ten points when their fructose intake is eliminated.

What follows with continued excess, daily fructose intake after the changes in our triglyceride and cholesterol profile and uric acid production can take a bit longer to develop. As we produce more abdominal fat, we become insulin resistant and are now predisposed to developing type 2 diabetes. This was known as adult-onset diabetes a few decades ago, but so many children have now acquired this metabolic derangement that it's referred to as type 2 diabetes. Type 1 diabetes is an autoimmune disorder, usually triggered by a viral illness, which leaves an individual insulin deficient. Type 2 diabetics have plenty of insulin; they're just resistant to its regulatory effects of our blood sugar levels. Consequently, type 1 diabetes isn't reversible, while type 2 diabetes can often be reversed by initiating appropriate diet and exercise changes (more on this later).

Sadly, the ravages of diabetes, kidney damage, high blood pressure, and gout can lead to significant suffering. But the ultimate outcome, now occurring in millions of Americans, is death due to stroke, heart attack, and kidney failure. This is a combination of fat imbalances (omega-3, omega-6) combined with the body damage metabolic syndrome causes. To date, the health care industry's response has been to use medications, dialysis, organ transplants, or operations on the heart and blood vessels at a cost of hundreds of billions of dollars per year. I've taken an aggressive approach with thousands of patients, since I've grown to understand metabolic syndrome. I've combined a multifaceted dietary change in affected individuals with amazing results. Many patients have seen a complete reversal of their metabolic derangements, a resolution of the inflammation damaging their bodies, and a decrease in abdominal fat deposition.

Let's return to the definition of metabolic syndrome before we proceed. Various definitions for metabolic syndrome have evolved from various countries, health organizations, and even the United Nations, with only a few variations. The commonly accepted definition in the United States is that we need to suffer from any three of five problems that include the following:

1. Elevated serum triglyceride
2. Reduced HDL cholesterol
3. High blood pressure
4. Type 2 diabetes
5. Increased abdominal girth

The first list I gave you above offers eight items. This list contains only five. The difference is that there are other changes that occur with the evolution of the metabolic syndrome in our bodies. The United States uses these five for the definition of metabolic syndrome, but some nations use different criteria to define it. Suffice it to say, we don't all manifest metabolic syndrome in the same way. In my practice as a gastroenterologist, I see fatty liver as an end product of fructose metabolism much more frequently than will a cardiologist who would see the heart manifestations. Your family physician may be managing your elevated cholesterol, high blood pressure, and obesity. Your endocrinologist may be trying to get your diabetes under control. Regardless, metabolic syndrome is a disorder that ends up affecting many organs because of the altered metabolism fructose excess causes.

An interesting aspect of fructose metabolism is that estrogen production in women helps to protect them against the belly fat aspect of metabolic syndrome. Once a woman loses her estrogen production, she will rapidly increase her waistline. If she stops consuming fructose, she will almost immediately begin to return to her former waistline. Additionally, some individuals don't become obese with daily excess fructose but can still manifest the metabolic syndrome without showing excess belly fat. The issue can also be a bit more complicated for some of us, as I will explain in the chapter concerning wheat and grains.

With production of triglyceride comes deposition of fat in our abdomens, but in many of us, it gets deposited in our liver as well. Over my lifetime as a physician, nonalcoholic fatty liver disease, as it is now known, has gone from a disease of obscurity to the number one cause of liver disease in America. The first case of fatty liver in children occurred in 1983, and it's now the primary liver disease seen in this age-group as well. The cause is primarily from excess daily fructose consumption, which leads to the metabolic syndrome.

I have witnessed dozens of medication treatment trials performed by academic physicians and funded by the pharmaceutical industry, with much failure. When I implemented the Lyons Lifestyle (the recommendations I describe in this book) and the patient was compliant, I witnessed a complete reversal of fatty liver. While the health care industry has been busy trying to treat symptoms or correct a lab value, I have tackled the problem of metabolic syndrome with patient education, implementation of dietary changes, and close monitoring with blood testing—with striking results. I presented my findings at a national meeting of the American College of Gastroenterology, but unfortunately, it's going to be some time before there's a change in the health care industry's approach to medical treatment. Many seek to reverse or control the disease process rather than prevent it in the first place. There are too many incentives for the present system to stay in place; there's too much money to be made on medicines and testing, and many are working against the preventive or reversal treatment approach of metabolic syndrome I ascribe to.

Let me make one last note about metabolic syndrome that isn't included in the definition but is clearly a manifestation of the progressive devastation seen in our bodies. This phenomenon is atrial fibrillation. This is an irregular fluttering of one's heartbeat that predisposes someone to sudden death with a rapid heart rate. It also leads to blood clots forming in our fibrillating heart chambers, leading to strokes. We now witness young people dropping dead in the sports arenas from no other apparent cause. My opinion is that these individuals perform their sports with an altered metabolism, which produces this sudden death. Autopsies don't reveal any other abnormalities in many of these individuals, and unfortunately, altered metabolism leading to atrial fibrillation cannot be detected in an autopsy.

Atrial fibrillation can also cause blood clots to form in the heart, which can then travel to the brain, legs, intestines, kidneys, and lungs. These blood clots can even kill you. Compound this problem with excessive omega-6 vegetable oil, which causes platelets to become sticky and promote blood clots, and again we have a perfect storm. Because of atrial fibrillation, patients are placed on blood thinners, which can then lead to intestinal bleeding, hospitalization, and death. The most common problem I see as a gastroenterologist, when I'm consulted for inpatient health issues, is intestinal bleeding caused by these blood thinners. If I perform a procedure that leads to an intestinal bleed, it's considered a complication from that procedure. If a patient develops an intestinal bleed from blood thinners, which were prescribed for atrial fibrillation caused by metabolic syndrome, we just accept it without questioning the cause. Often too much fructose is the cause.

The most recent recommendation of the Food and Drug Administration for high blood pressure in America is to reduce salt intake and decrease the amount of salt in processed foods. While I'm not against prudent salt reduction in our diets, reducing excess fructose prevents the cause of high blood pressure in the first place. Decreasing salt intake helps to treat the symptom, but to prevent high blood pressure in the first place, a by-product of metabolic syndrome, we must eliminate the excessive fructose driving this process.

We need to become educated about metabolic syndrome. We need to understand how it affects us. We can stop the damage occurring throughout our bodies in a multitude of ways. We can prevent irreversible affects that eventually develop. We need to attack the cause rather than just treat the effects with pills, stents, and surgeries. We need to stop premature death witnessed daily across America. We can dramatically reduce needless suffering and premature death if we stop consuming excess fructose from fruit, juices, honey, high-fructose corn syrup, and table sugar (including organic agave syrup) every day.

Pearls

- Daily, excessive fructose consumption causes metabolic syndrome.
- Seventy million American adults and millions of our youth currently suffer from metabolic syndrome.
- Metabolic syndrome leads to premature death from atrial fibrillation, heart disease, and stroke, cirrhosis from fatty liver, kidney disease, and so forth.
- Metabolic syndrome is preventable or reversible in nearly all of us with appropriate dietary changes.

CHAPTER 6

Gluten

Do not bite at the bait of pleasure, till you
know there is no hook beneath it.

Thomas Jefferson

If we watch a baker toss dough into the air and shape a pizza over his or her outstretched arm and hand, we will notice its amazing elasticity. As the kneading proceeds by massaging the pizza crust farther and farther into a thinner and larger crust, we marvel that the baker doesn't shred the dough and that it doesn't fall apart. Is this event due to the amazing talent of the pizza pie maker or the special properties of the dough?

What allows this process to occur is a substance found in the dough, called "gluten." This protein was a foreign term to most of us just a few years ago, but today nearly everyone has heard about it. Whether it's in the context of "gluten allergy," "gluten free," or "gluten intolerance," most of us are familiar with gluten to some degree. I want to educate you about gluten and explain why it has caused significant problems to millions of us in just a few short decades.

Gluten is a protein found primarily in wheat, barley, and rye. It's naturally found in small quantities in other grains as well, but the primary source in America is wheat. Over the last several decades, genetic hybridization of wheat has led to an increased concentration of gluten in wheat. Some reports claim that there is as much gluten in a single slice of bread today as was present in forty to one hundred slices of bread in 1960.

The consequence of excess gluten consumption is now showing its ugly face. Some of us cannot tolerate the excess amount of gluten found in the many processed foods we consume. We are exposed to it in breads, cakes, cookies, pancakes, waffles, bagels, pastas, muffins, pie crusts, rolls, hamburger and hotdog buns, pretzels, and crackers of all types. We see it added to foods as a flavor and texture enhancer; we find it in cosmetics, hair treatments, and skin products; and we find it in protein supplements. We find it cross contaminated in the milling of gluten-free grains, such as oats.

This markedly increased exposure to gluten has led to a number of medical problems in some of us. The most devastating outcome has been the rise of a disease known as celiac disease. This is a disorder caused by gluten exposure to the intestinal lining, which leads to an immunologic reaction. What follows is variable in any of us, but it can manifest itself as abdominal pain, bloating, diarrhea, or malabsorption. The malabsorption can, in turn, lead to anemia, osteoporosis, skin problems, hair loss, altered mental state, and the like. Long-term, untreated celiac disease can lead to incurable intestinal cancers and lymphoma.

The incidence of celiac disease has increased 300 percent since the 1940s. While it's a genetically predisposed disorder in many people, it is now being diagnosed in individuals who don't express the genetic risk factor. Many of us are unaware that we have celiac disease and can go undiagnosed for years. The consequences can be devastating in many of us if the disease isn't managed appropriately.

Not everyone who is sensitive to gluten suffers from celiac disease; regardless, we can still feel the consequences of excess gluten. Some of us may have gastrointestinal distress in various forms, including excess gas, bloating, nausea and/or vomiting, intestinal cramping, altered bowel habits, constipation, or diarrhea. Others may suffer from headaches, seizures, anxiety, ADHD, dementia, schizophrenia, Parkinson's disease, depression, autism, muscle twitching (such as shaky leg syndrome), delayed childhood growth, infertility, or miscarriages. Two excellent books, recently published concerning the effects of gluten, are *Wheat Belly* by Dr. William Davis and *Grain Brain* by Dr. David Perlmutter. Rather than trying to repeat all the data found in these excellent volumes, I would encourage you to read them if you want to delve into this topic more deeply. Suffice it to say, gluten intolerance plays a major role in many who suffer from these and other medical conditions.

When we eat food, our brains talk to our intestinal tracts through numerous hormones to regulate hunger and stimulate the feeling that we are "full" after consuming a meal. As we learned in the chapter about fructose, when fructose is consumed, it alters blood flow in the brain to overstimulate hunger. Consequently, we continue to feel hungry, even though our stomachs may be full. Gluten also affects the brain in a negative way. This protein tells our brains that we aren't full. Isn't it ironic? One component says, "Feed me," and the other says, "Don't stop" feeding me. No wonder overeating in America has resulted in our obesity problem.

I wrote an exhaustive paper about gluten and celiac disease. It is posted on my website: http://www.lyonsmedicalnews.com. I would encourage you to read it sometime. While it contains lots of medical terms, it will enlighten you to many facts I haven't included in this chapter.

I don't believe it's essential for most of us to give up all forms of gluten, as we have the capacity to enjoy foods that contain this protein without the dire consequences seen in celiac disease if we do so properly. I also know, though, that if you suffer from the many symptoms an overexposure to gluten can cause or trigger, it would be worth your time to ask your physician to test you to see whether you are forming antibodies to gluten. Some of us just feel better on a low-gluten or gluten-free diet, even if we don't form those antibodies.

Gluten isn't a necessary component in our diets to maintain nutritional health, but it can lead to a rather restrictive diet. Many grocery stores now have a gluten-free section that has expanded with the growing demand from consumers. Gluten-free products are often more expensive than gluten-laden foods. Regardless, my feeling is that, if we have symptoms that don't have an apparent cause, it may be worth a dietary trial to see whether gluten negatively affects us. Repeat challenges may be required on your part to make this determination. One thing to remember about gluten intolerance, though, is that it may take three to six months to truly see a change, since the damage gluten causes can take months for our bodies to repair.

Gluten is also found in other grains, such as bulgur, spelt, and couscous. It is found in some beers, condiments, many processed foods, and additives. When in doubt, check it out. Foods such as rice, potatoes, quinoa, corn, and soy are considered gluten free. In processing they can become contaminated, and presently there is no defined regulation on the food label concerning gluten content. Producers will label something "gluten free" as an enticement to get people to consume the product, but the Food and Drug Administration mandates that the statement be true.

The next time you bite into that soft, chewy pizza after it got tossed into the air to be stretched before entering the brick oven, you now understand that this process is allowed because of gluten. This protein brings pleasure to our gastronomic endeavors. For those of us who love pizza, pasta, or a Reuben sandwich, gluten enhances that experience. We just need to remember not to indulge in excess of omega-6 fat, fructose, and now gluten.

Pearls

- Gluten is a protein found primarily in wheat, barley, and rye grains.
- Gluten content in wheat has increased dramatically in the past fifty years.
- Gluten can cause many medical problems, including celiac disease.
- Celiac disease has increased 300 percent in America since the 1940s.
- Excess gluten may cause many symptoms: be aware.

CHAPTER 7

Limit Wheat and Refined Grains

The goal of education is the advancement of
knowledge and the dissemination of truth.
John F. Kennedy

I was recently watching a 1962 James Bond movie, and the "advanced" gadgetry Mr. Bond displayed while saving the world amused me. Rotary phones, fancy race cars, a personal jet pack to fly an individual (Mr. Bond) from a rooftop to avoid capture, and a cigarette that functioned as a gun are some of the now archaic relics of that era. If you watch a modern Bond movie, the acrobatics, electronic gadgetry, phones, computer technology, and the like have dramatically changed as well. But the plot is always the same: Mr. Bond must save the world from destruction, but the methods, "action toys," and acrobatics have advanced with the times.

If you were to look at a slice of bread from 1962, you would find a very simple wheat flour kneaded into the dough, which makes up your peanut butter and jelly sandwich. Then along came Wonder Bread, which was soft and spongy, and the rave for all kids to enjoy. The lightness was due to the addition of gluten, which made its texture so superior to typical breads of its day; the bread was much more appealing to all of us (see previous chapter). What also began to occur with wheat was that hybridization and genetic modification of wheat began to transform the plant and grain into a high-yield, short-stalked plant. This change led to a massive increase in wheat production unlike America had ever seen.

This grain crop contained nearly twenty times the yield of just a decade earlier in the 1950s. The grain was packed full of gluten and sugars. Over the next two decades, because of an abundance of grain crops, we saw a transformation of foodstuffs that stocked our supermarket shelves, restaurants, and fast-food chains. A hamburger bun increased in size from less than one hundred calories to over two hundred. The typical meal tripled in size and caloric intake.

Another major change that occurred as we were dramatically altering our intake of wheat was the massive effort by U.S. Government agencies, agribusiness, and Big Pharma to get us to believe that America's health was deteriorating because of cholesterol and saturated fats. We had been consuming these forms of fat from farm foods for centuries until the powers of centralized government (Health and Human Services, Food and Drug Administration, Department of Agriculture, and National Institute of Health), academic nutrition, and big business began convincing us that the cause of the massive explosion of heart disease and cancer was saturated fats and cholesterol in our diets rather than trans fat consumption, omega-6 fat excess, and other causes.

In 1958 our federal government was provided data that trans fats were the primary culprit of the rapid rise in deaths related to cancer and heart disease. Corporate America needed a scapegoat to divert our attention away from this fact, so they engaged in a massive lobbying campaign to promote the idea that cows, eggs, and other sources of farm fats were the cause. They advanced the idea that the natural alternative food source for protein and calories that needed to replace the foods that had been meeting our nutritional needs for millennia was wheat. The increased demand for wheat and other grains led to a shift from a high-protein, high-fat diet to the high-carbohydrate, low-fat diet. This has been the centerpiece of the American diet for the past sixty years. We're now suffering with the medical consequences of those changes.

Wheat is packed full of a sugar that is different from fructose. That sugar is a unique form of glucose known as amylopectin. When we hear the word *starch*, potatoes and rice immediately come to mind. Our blood sugar is glucose, and when our pancreas enzymes digest starch or amylopectin, glucose is released and absorbed into our bloodstream. Once the glucose is in the bloodstream, one of three events then occurs.

The first event that happens is a rapid rise in blood sugar, which directly leads to energy production in the forms of ATP (adenosine triphosphate; the primary molecule that provides energy to our cells) and other energy molecules. These forms of energy then allow our muscles to work; they allow production of enzymes, antibodies, new cells, and so forth.

The second event that can occur with this precipitous influx of glucose in our veins is its storage in our livers or muscles as glycogen. The body has a unique emergency battery system to supply us with glucose on demand, and that battery is glycogen. Let's say we get up in the morning and go for a two-mile run before breakfast. We begin our workout, and our muscles start to demand glucose to meet the demands of pushing our feet down the trail. As soon as our blood sugar drops, the glycogen battery is called on to release the stored glucose to feed our lungs, hearts, and muscles. If glycogen isn't released, we would rapidly become hypoglycemic and suffer symptoms of light-headedness, cold clamminess, weakness, confusion, seizures, coma, and even death if blood sugars continue to fall too much.

The glycogen battery is necessary for our bodies to function well. But the glycogen battery is also limited. This takes us to the third event that happens after we've eaten our wheat or starch product. If blood sugar levels are adequate and the glycogen battery is full, the excess glucose is converted to fat and placed in long-term storage in our fat cells. Our bodies have the ability to move fat in and out of our cells and to have it converted to glucose if we've emptied the glycogen battery. If we chronically keep our glycogen batteries empty, our bodies' chemistry switches to a fatty acid energy system (kind of like an alternative energy source in a hybrid car). This is what occurs with marathon runners, long-distance bicyclists, swimmers, and triathlon competitors. Because they routinely exceed their glycogen battery during their athletic endeavors, they rely on fat conversion for energy. This is the reason why these individuals typically have a low percentage of body fat. Most of us aren't so fortunate. Interestingly, this glucose-starved state is the principle behind the Atkins and other low-carbohydrate diets.

What has happened to most of us is that we've transformed our bodies into fat-storage machines rather than primarily living off our glycogen batteries. Several mechanisms cause this to occur, and I'll try to keep this as comprehensible as possible without getting too technical.

A typical meal size has increased by several hundred calories per day since 1970. When I was in high school, a box of popcorn would hold less than the scoop that fills the tubs of popcorn we consume today. A typical hamburger was about 350 calories; the giant burgers we enjoy today are at least one thousand calories or more. The volume of a soda pop has grown from ten ounces to twenty ounces or more (and all the free refills you can drink at your favorite restaurant). A family-size pizza of the 1970 era is now considered a small pie. I could go on, but you get the picture. We're eating much larger servings today. This fact keeps our glycogen battery overfilled, and calories are passed into fat storage.

Second, we eat more wheat products, and the starch is making changes to our metabolism. If you eat a piece of any kind of meat or egg, you won't see much of a change in your blood sugar. When you consume wheat products, however, that sugar is rapidly digested and causes the highest spike in your blood sugar of any food you eat.

Without making this too scientific, let me say that this sugar spike causes your body's hormones to drive that excess sugar into your fat storage, bypassing your glycogen battery.

The third event is that your brain is convinced that you're hungry, even though you've just consumed hundreds, if not thousands, of calories. The effects of gluten and other wheat proteins directly on the brain have caused this. The rapid change in our blood sugar, caused by the wheat starch intake, leads to feeling hungry as soon as that blood sugar level comes crashing back down.

Another consequence of consuming wheat is the effect on vitamin D metabolism. Studies now document that wheat metabolism directly leads to vitamin D deficiency. We now see that millions of Americans suffer the consequences of vitamin D deficiency with osteoporosis, autoimmune diseases, heart disease, depression, and chronic fatigue. Sunshine is a major source of vitamin D renewal in our bodies, but we've increased our consumption of wheat by 30 percent, from 113 pounds to 146 pounds per person per year, since 1970. In that same time period, we've seen massive increases in the diseases associated with vitamin D deficiency. The vitamin D deficiency story is complicated, so I will discuss it in its own chapter.

America's health care industry's response has been to develop new drugs to treat osteoporosis and replace failing joints, supplement our diets with vitamin D pills, and increase the use of health care by billions of dollars per year. At the same time the food pyramid and now the MyPlate guidelines US government agencies and agribusiness provide strongly encourage us to consume more wheat products.

Two grains that have been part the diet of Central and South America for millennia are chia and quinoa, respectively. Their popularity has grown in the United States in the past few years, as people are looking for alternative grains to wheat. As word has spread about the harmful effects of genetically modified wheat, excess gluten, and metabolic disasters (which have been written about in the books

I referenced above), vegetarians, vegans, and concerned omnivores are aggressively looking for alternatives.

Both grains are excellent sources of omega-3 fat, high-density protein, and vitamins and minerals. They both contain quite a bit of carbohydrates, and quinoa has sixty-four grams of sugars per serving and ten times more omega-6 fat than omega-3 fat. As you can see, if you add this to an already-bloated intake of fructose in your diet, you may actually compound the problems related to fructose and metabolic syndrome. If you've been able to shut down this problem, then these gluten-free grains are an excellent alternative to wheat, barley, and rye. But use them sparingly, since they contain excessive carbohydrates, which can maintain metabolic syndrome if fructose has activated this problem. It's in the balance of fats, sugars, and grains that we can optimize our metabolism and health.

Pearls

- Wheat and grains contain excess sugars that are harmful to our health if we consume too many servings per day.
- Excess grain consumption leads or contributes to diabetes, metabolic syndrome, obesity, vitamin D deficiency, gluten-related problems, and so forth.
- Sugars found in grains compound the effects of excess fructose metabolism.
- Consume grains sparingly rather than as a mainstay to your diet.

CHAPTER 8

The Obesity Epidemic

The learning and knowledge that we have, is, at the most,
but little compared with that of which we are ignorant.

Plato

When I attended high school, very few of us were overweight, let alone morbidly obese. I was one of the bigger kids in my graduating class, weighing 170 pounds and rising six foot one. In today's world, I would be considered skinny, yet I had no concept at the time that others would now look at me and think of me as being a lean young man. If you look at a typical high school senior class today, at least 17 percent of the graduates are obese, and 32 percent are considered overweight.

A recently released study showed that over one billion people worldwide are now obese. America is one of the leaders of expanding waistlines but isn't yet leading the world, since Mexico is number one. Two out of every three adults in the United States are now overweight or obese. The number of affected people has tripled in my lifetime. The explosion of our waistlines began to occur in the late 1970s. Fortunately or unfortunately, the percentage of adults affected by excess weight has now hit a plateau at 68 percent. The problem is that we aren't getting smaller. For the first time in American history, we now have about four million people who weigh over three hundred pounds, and nearly a half million weigh over four hundred pounds.

What has changed in the last forty years? As I discussed earlier, we're definitely eating larger portions. Meal size is about 35 percent bigger now than in 1970. We also consume excessive amounts of grains, sugars, snack foods, soda pop, fruit, and juices compared to the time before our waistlines began to expand.

There isn't just one culprit to blame for the enlarging of America. As I pointed out in the fructose and wheat chapters, we now consume much more of both. Fructose metabolism alters our chemistry to cause the metabolic syndrome. This leads to what is known as "central obesity" that manifests itself as excess belly fat and increased abdominal girth. This type of obesity is very dangerous, since it predisposes us to heart disease and stroke.

Wheat and other grains and starches produce excess calories leading to global obesity. It had been known for years that pear-shaped bodies (big behinds and thighs) didn't predispose one to heart disease, but excess weight caused a breakdown of weight-bearing joints.

Today we now suffer from both problems: global (total body) and central (belly fat) obesity. Central obesity occurs from daily, excess fructose metabolism; and peripheral, pear-shaped obesity comes from too many calories from excess carbohydrate intake derived from wheat, grains, and other starch sources as well as too many total calories from other food groups. We are now plagued on two fronts. We've increased fresh fruit consumption by almost 30 percent, sweetener use (table sugar and high-fructose corn syrup) by 39 percent, and grains (wheat, corn, and rice) by over 40 percent. At the same time, we've decreased our egg consumption (saturated fat) by 35 percent, potato consumption (starch) by 25 percent, and red meat consumption (protein and saturated fat) by 20 percent. Interestingly, we've increased fish consumption (protein, saturated fat, and omega-3 fat) by almost 50 percent.

As you can see, it's difficult to point the finger at just one food based on these numbers. More importantly, it's imperative to understand what our bodies do with excess calories. By now, you realize that not all consumed calories are equal. We've increased our overall total caloric intake by about 25 percent. Most calories have come from fruit, sweeteners, and grains. The rest has come from vegetable oils and olive oil. While we decreased our overall fat intake, which has more calories per ounce than sugars, we dramatically increased our carbohydrate intake.

When you place your key into the ignition switch of your car and turn the key, you expect it to start right up. The reason you rely on this to occur is because there is a battery of stored energy that, when released by the starter switch, causes the engine to turn over and begin to run of its own accord. Most automobiles have only one battery system, but the human body is unique in that we have *two* battery systems to get us out of bed, perform mental processes, and go for a five-kilometer run before our morning shower. Our battery system has two supplies we draw on, depending on the nature and duration of the activity, the type and amount of food we consume, our underlying health state, and other factors I won't go into here.

What's important to understand is that the primary energy source in a car battery is stored electricity, while in our bodies; our immediate source of energy expenditure is derived from blood glucose. As our blood sugar level starts to fall, our bodies mobilize more sugar stored in the form of glycogen from our red blood cells, muscles, and liver (and to a lesser degree in other organs). Glycogen is a large compound of many glucose molecules tightly packed together, which can then be broken back down to form freely circulating glucose when our blood sugar levels begin to fall. In the plant kingdom, we find stored glucose in the form of starch (potatoes, rice, and so forth) and amylopectin (grains).

The body has a limited capacity to store glucose in this glycogen battery. For most of us, this is a fixed amount, but we can increase the size of our glycogen battery with vigorous exercise. When we eat carbohydrates, the absorbed sugars promptly cause our blood level of glucose to rise. Our insulin kicks in and stimulates the formation of glycogen in the various storage sites in the above mentioned organs. Once this battery is completely filled and the body has excess sugar to store, this leads to another set of chemical reactions. The glucose is converted to fat in the form of triglyceride and is placed in the fat battery. The fat battery functions as a long-term storage battery, while the glycogen battery is the daily backup battery for a source of energy. Only when you've emptied your glycogen battery will your body call on your fat battery to meet your metabolic needs. Alternatively, if you don't consume carbohydrates regularly, your body has the uncanny ability to switch to the long-term battery and live off your stored fat for immediate energy.

High-power athletes learned this fact some time ago and avoid carbohydrates for this very reason. A great insight about this is documented in the recently published book *The Boys in the Boat* by Daniel James Brown. This is the gripping story of nine young men from the University of Washington who overcame multiple forms of adversity to win the 1936 Berlin Olympics in eight-oar crew. This story is the epitome of carbohydrate avoidance at its finest. The coach was a strict dietary disciplinarian since he knew carbohydrates severely hamper peak performance.

As Nina Teicholz points out in her new book *The Big Fat Surprise,* the long-held myth of "carbohydrate loading" prior to athletic competition has been debunked. Studies reveal that competitors have reduced performances when they rely on their sugar batteries for energy rather than on their fat batteries. Additionally, these superstar participants have a very low body mass of fat.

In the past fifty years, America has become a high carbohydrate-consuming nation. We've given up a diet of protein and high-quality fat, and we're now daily filling our diets with massive quantities of carbohydrates. Our carbohydrate intake now accounts for up to 75 percent of our caloric needs if we adhere to the MyPlate nutritional guidelines the federal government has provided. This occurs in the form of fruits, juices, honey, sugar, and high-fructose corn syrup. It includes crackers, cookies, cakes, cupcakes, waffles, pancakes, bagels, muffins, smoothies, ice cream, candies, breads, hamburger buns, hotdog buns, biscuits, potato chips, corn chips, french fries, tortillas, pastas, pastries, French toast, cold cereals loaded with sugars, pizza, calzones, sandwiches, croissants, yogurts loaded with fruit, and sweeteners. The list seems endless in today's diet choices.

When I was a kid, we typically ate a meat, vegetable, and potatoes meal. It was a rare occasion when the meal ventured beyond this typical approach to dining. Additionally, a peanut butter and jelly sandwich consisted of wheat that had yet to undergo genetic modification to contain the massive quantities of sugar (amylopectin) and gluten today's varieties are loaded with. Breakfast was typically a bowl of hot oatmeal or a couple of eggs in the winter and perhaps a bowl of oat, corn, or rice cereal in the summertime. We enjoyed homemade pie on Sunday afternoons and a tart apple after school. We even had a cookie on occasion. But the sugar load was so much less than it is today. Fructose intake alone has increased 850 percent from 1960 to the present time. That doesn't even account for all the other sugars in the other products we consume daily today.

The outcome of this massive increase in our carbohydrate intake is that our glycogen battery is always full unless we're quite vigorous in our physical activity. We're continuously adding to our fat battery. What's worse is that the type of obesity we're seeing today is central obesity. This is the fat deposition in our abdomens, which occurs as a consequence of the metabolic syndrome. It has been known for decades that if you were big in the hips, buttocks, and thighs, you were just fat; but that condition didn't have much of an impact on your health other than an excess burden on your weight-bearing joints and spine.

Unfortunately, the abdominal obesity we see in epidemic proportions is the type of excess weight associated with numerous medical problems. These conditions will cause significant morbidity, and ultimately it will shorten one's life expectancy.

I pointed out in the chapter on metabolic syndrome that all the diseases discussed there are associated with abdominal obesity, so I won't repeat that discussion here. It's important to point out, though, that other disorders occur because of this kind of obesity. These include male hypogonadism, gynecomastia (breast enlargement), menstrual irregularities, polycystic ovarian syndrome, and female hirsutism (excess female facial hair). Central obesity is also associated with sleep apnea, snoring, and pulmonary hypertension. It's also present with fatty liver disease, cirrhosis of the liver, gastroesophageal reflux disease, and gallstones.

The worst complication related to central obesity is cancer. In men, cancer of the esophagus, colon, rectum, pancreas, liver, and prostate are all significantly increased in those affected by central obesity. In women, cancer of the gallbladder, liver, esophagus, breast, cervix, ovary, uterus, and bile duct have all been reported in this scenario. The most recent estimates of cancer deaths related to central obesity are 14 percent for men and 20 percent for women.

The obesity epidemic has yet to plateau in America. While the baby boomer generation seems to have leveled out at around 68 percent of the population, our young people are now joining in on the fat growth.

Obesity is now spreading across the world, since many cultures have begun to abandon their native diets in favor of the carbohydrate-rich Western diet of the United States. Many Asian, African, and Central and South American countries have seen a steady rise in central obesity and its associated diseases in recent decades. The native people of Greenland are one very prominent example. Up until the past twenty years or so, there was virtually no diabetes or heart disease among them. In that country, they consumed a high-protein, high-fat diet with almost no carbohydrates. They have now incorporated carbohydrates in the form of grain products and sweets into their old diets, and various diseases are now on the rise.

Those in the Mediterranean region and much of Europe have refused to adopt our high-carbohydrate, low-fat diet; and their progress toward obesity has occurred much more slowly. They consume a high-protein, high-fat (especially fish and olive oil) diet with vegetables and old-world grains that haven't been genetically modified or hybridized. Consequently, they have a diet that is very similar to the diet of my youth, with the exception of farm fats rather than olive oil. The incidence of diseases there is lower than in America if they haven't switched over to the low-fat, high-carbohydrate, trans-fats-rich, vegetable-oil-rich diets we consume.

The French paradox, a diet high in saturated fats (primarily butter) and protein but low in carbohydrates, has been the discussion of the Food and Drug Administration and the academic circles of American medicine for decades. The French diet is atypical for a "Mediterranean" diet, yet those in this diet also have a low incidence of heart disease while consuming many more saturated fats than we do. They are spared obesity and many of the diseases that plague us. As I point out in the next chapter on saturated fats, obesity isn't caused by these fats but by a high-carbohydrate, low-fat diet.

We adopted the food pyramid in the early 1990's after the US Department of Agriculture spent years refining an educational approach to promote nutritional health for America. A massive educational campaign was put into place from those in kindergarten to college in an attempt to get us to change our diets. The food pyramid encouraged us to consume six to eleven servings of grains, three to six servings of vegetables, and two to three servings of fruit per day. It persuaded us to eat three times as many carbohydrates as in previous generations.

In 2010, we changed from the food pyramid to the MyPlate

guidelines in an attempt to again move toward a healthier diet. This diet plan recommends that we consume three-quarters of our meal with carbohydrates. This is divided fairly equally between grains, fruits, and vegetables. As you've learned, if we eat this many carbohydrates, we will become obese and alter our metabolism. What is worse, obesity begins to develop as a young child and is perpetuated throughout life when we follow this diet plan. Our bodies cannot process this many sugar calories and continue to maintain health.

We need to make a concerted effort to dramatically reduce our fat battery as a nation and increase our physical activity to enlarge our glycogen battery so the excess sugar we consume doesn't spill over into fat. We also need to dramatically decrease our carbohydrate intake of fruits, grains, and other sweetened products on a daily basis so we don't chronically add to our fat batteries. To the contrary, we're being advised to daily consume three servings of fruit and several servings of grains. This practice will chronically surpass our glycogen battery and add to our fat battery unless we're involved in vigorous athletic activities. This diet also alters our metabolism so these sugars preferentially get stored as fat if we consume them in excess for as little as two consecutive weeks (see my book *Fructose Exposed*).

Here's one final thought concerning carbohydrate intake and obesity. If you chronically consume very few carbohydrates, I recommend that you pick one treat day every seven to ten days and eat all the carbohydrates your heart desires on that particular day. Studies show that a single day of carbohydrate indulgence doesn't hurt your metabolism and actually temporarily increases your metabolic rate. That is a good thing, and you will get the psychological pleasure of enjoying that plate of brownies or bag of M&M's. Just don't make every day a treat day.

By the way, very few vegetables count as carbohydrates, since they have very few sugars present. The biggest exceptions are sugar beets, sweet corn, sweet peas, and sweet potatoes, as their names imply. It's best to consume these on your treat day if you're dying to enjoy one or all of them.

If you're quite athletic and exercise at least an hour per day, you can probably tolerate up to one hundred grams of carbohydrates per day, but for most of us, who work in a sedentary job at a desk and might be fortunate to average thirty to forty-five minutes of exercise per day, our sugar load should be closer to twenty to thirty grams of carbohydrates (ten to fifteen grams of fructose) per day. Many of us cannot tolerate too many sugar calories, because our intestines react negatively with bloating, cramping, and altering bowel habits when we overindulge. You must find your comfort zone, but you need to know that the reason we're getting fat is because of carbohydrates, not protein and fat consumption.

Pearls

- Obesity now affects two-thirds of adults and one-third of the youth in America.
- The cause of obesity has many causes.
- The primary cause of obesity is excess, daily consumption of carbohydrates (fruits, sugars, and grains).
- Most of us need to limit our carbohydrate intake to about twenty to thirty grams (ten to fifteen grams of fructose) per day to prevent obesity.

CHAPTER 9

Don't Worry about Saturated Fats

There are no constraints on the human mind, no
walls around the human spirit, no barriers to our
progress except those we ourselves erect.
Ronald Reagan

Before the discovery of vitamins and their importance in the
causation of diseases in the first half of the twentieth century, no
one really cared about vitamins. Once scientists elucidated these vital
protein-like compounds, we were then educated about these substances
and their importance in maintaining health. Prior to our new found
education, we were none the wiser about the existence of vitamins,
their importance, or our lack of education about these substances,
which were sustaining us. Most of us now know the significance of
vitamins, but at the time of their discovery, we acquired most of our
vitamins from a glass of milk or a fried egg, vegetables, or some other
unadulterated farm food. As long as we consumed these and other
nutritious foods on a regular basis, we were nutritionally replete.

Much of the same can be said for saturated fats. Up until the
1950s, we had grown up consuming saturated fats in the form of farm
animal fats, wild game, fish, coconut oil, palm oil, and the like. But

then along came a study published early in that decade that suggested that consumption of saturated fats from animal fats was the cause of the exploding rise of heart disease across America, which developed after World War II. The problem with this information was that it contradicted how we'd been living without heart disease for centuries. But somehow nobody seemed to adequately question the conclusion of the study or a second investigation by the same university investigator four years later. Instead, the federal government (National Institutes of Health and Food and Drug Administration), academic nutrition, and the American Heart Association launched an educational blitz to get us off saturated fats.

What I'm trying to get you to understand about saturated fats goes opposite, until very recently, of teachings of every major medical organization and government agency as it relates to these fats. As a matter of fact, it's remarkable that this push to change the American diet occurred at all because there was a major flaw in the study on which this movement was based.

When Dr. Ancel Keys of the University of Minnesota published his "six" country study about saturated fats, there appeared to be a linear relationship between the increasing consumption of saturated fats and the increased frequency of heart disease. The problem arises in the fact that he excluded all the countries (sixteen to be exact) in his analysis that contradicted his thesis. When other researchers analyzed all the data, there was absolutely no correlation, let alone a cause and effect, seen between saturated fats and heart disease.

Four years later, he then published his "seven country" study, which supported his first study. Again, he threw out all data that didn't support his thesis, which were about 90 percent of the data. At the same time, he was able to convince many people in positions that controlled the purse strings for research that, based on his findings, it was necessary to change the American diet. He blackballed anyone who didn't get on board with his thesis. He and others who joined his cause were able to turn off research grants to those who opposed his thinking. They blocked publication of data that contradicted him; they ostracized researchers from national science meetings; and they established policies in academic, federal, and political circles that made saturated fats leprous. If you're interested in reading the entire historical account of how this all occurred, I highly recommend Nina Teicholz's *New York Times* bestseller, *The Big Fat Surprise*.

We've now been "educated" for nearly three generations that saturated fats will cause us to develop heart disease, and we've seen a massive decline in the consumption of these fats since the 1960s. In spite of the dietary decline of saturated fat intake and the increase of low-saturated-fat consumption of skim milk, 1 percent or 2 percent milk, low-fat cheeses, fat-free yogurts, nonfat half-and-half, yolkless eggs, fat-free ice cream, and on and on, we've witnessed a steady and rapid rise in heart disease. While we decreased our egg and red meat intake, we witnessed an explosion and ever-increasing number of people suffering from the very diseases we were told these saturated-fat-laden foods caused. All the changes to the Western diet to get us on a low-saturated-fat, high-carbohydrate diet have failed miserably when it comes to reducing heart attacks, strokes, and peripheral vascular disease.

Let me explain why this is the case by demonstrating what saturated fats are and what their function in our bodies is. I know most people aren't biology or chemistry majors, but I think there are some concepts nearly all of us understand. First, our bodies are made up of billions of cells. Those cells have a membrane that keeps the inside cell contents in and the outside contents out. Without the membrane, the cell would die, and we wouldn't be able to stay alive. This is true of all living plant and animal life. Our cell membranes are composed primarily of fats. While the composition of different cell membranes varies from one type of cell to the next, the most important fats found in these membranes are saturated fats. Without these fats in our cell membranes, our cells would be weakened to the point of leaking out vital contents of the cells, and they would be increasingly vulnerable to substances outside the cell gaining access to the inside of the cell. This would cause damage and death to the cell.

Saturated fats don't mix with water. If you add some bacon grease to water, you can readily see this truth. These same saturated fats keep excess water out of a cell and water content inside the cell stable. Roughly half of the fats found in cell membranes are saturated fats. It's safe to say that without these fats, life as we know and understand it couldn't exist.

Saturated fats have been consumed for millennia. They come in the form of farm and wild animal fats (lard, tallow, butterfat, and egg yolk) and plant fats (palm, coconut, palm kernel, and dark chocolate). In the last half of the twentieth century, we've dramatically decreased their use in our diets. We've supplanted them with vegetable oils rich in omega-6 fat and manufactured trans fats. When the government and the medical industry started the push to reduce intake of saturated fats in the 1950s, manufactured trans fats had already been incorporated into our diets, and omega-6-rich (inflammatory) vegetable oil consumption was on the rise.

Ironically, the federal government deems olive oil as heart healthy. Olive oil is rich in omega-9 fat known as oleic acid. Our livers convert omega-9 fat to saturated fat when our cells signal the liver for their production. So a precursor to saturated fats is healthy, but saturated fats aren't? This is an oxymoron, to say the least. Chemistry tells us one thing; the Food and Drug Administration tells us another.

Beyond maintaining the integrity of cell membranes, massive amounts of scientific data now reveal the importance of saturated fats in many other parts of our bodies. While I'm not going to list every benefit, it's important to realize that the brain, bones, liver, heart, lungs, kidneys, and hormone health are directly tied to adequate saturated fat consumption. Data also now abundantly show the importance of saturated fats in maintaining strong cell-to-cell communication, a healthy immune system and the prevention of obesity. The irony is that manufactured trans fats and omega-6-rich vegetable oils block many of the functions saturated fats perform in our bodies.

In the past three decades, dozens of studies have been published, vindicating the importance and safety of saturated fats. Several recent meta-analyses (a method of analyzing several studies concerning the same topic being questioned in an attempt to derive a common or divergent answer) have all come to the same conclusion. Saturated fats aren't the cause of heart disease or stroke. Yet major health organizations—such as the American Heart Association; the American Dietetic Association; and government agencies such as the Department of Health and Human Services, the Centers for Disease Control, the Food and Drug Administration, and the World Health Organization—all continue to recommend the reduction of saturated fats in our diets. What's more, the food label lumps saturated fats with manufactured trans fats. As you learned in the trans fat chapter, the federal government allows the food industry to conceal the quantity of trans fat in our food and then confuses us further by discouraging us from eating a fat (saturated fat) that is important to multiple aspects of nutritional health.

Clearly there are incentives at play here that would cause many health organizations and government agencies to all support reduction of saturated fats from our diets, while mountains of data contradict this conclusion. Additionally, the original conclusions by Dr. Ancel Keys concerning saturated fat and heart disease have now been proved to be falsified information. Bringing pressure on legislators and food manufacturers is going to be necessary to reverse this alarming practice when it isn't in the best interests of the public. Those knowingly promoting poor health practices need to be held accountable.

Many populations around the world consume a diet rich in saturated fats and do not suffer from heart disease or many other medical conditions seen in the western world from consuming a high carbohydrate, low saturated fat diet. People such as the Maasai and Samburu Indians of Africa consume over a half pound of butterfat (very high in saturated fat) daily, yet they don't die from heart disease. It's only when they give up their native high-saturated fat diet and consume a Western diet that they develop heart disease. The same phenomenon has been documented among the Polynesians, Arctic Inuit, and Greenland Eskimos.

I would encourage all of us to keep an open mind about saturated fats. We must relearn common sense about these fats. All our ancestors lived on them without getting the diseases we suffer from today. Several populations on the planet currently live on these fats without the influence of the West, and they live healthy lives.

Scientific studies too voluminous to recount in this chapter contradict health organizations and government agency recommendations. While I don't have a concrete answer for this dichotomy between scientific fact and public policy, I think it's safe to say that my advice to you concerning the consumption of saturated fats is sound. Don't be fearful of keeping saturated fats in your diet. The more closely those fats are consumed in relationship to the way nature produced them is best.

Hybridization, genetic modification of grains and fruits, hydrogenation of omega-6-rich vegetable oils, and altered diets of farm animals all have an impact on the composition of the foods we eat. These changes to our food products can affect the beneficial effects of some foods. If you feed a chicken cornmeal, the composition of the egg and meat will be different than if the chicken is allowed to roam around the yard to find food or if it is fed flax meal. One diet is rich in omega-6 fats, while the other is rich to omega-3 fats. The saturated fat content remains the same with either diet. Likewise, pasteurization and homogenization of milk destroy the integrity of omega-3 and saturated fats in milk, so we lose the natural benefit of these fats compared to unprocessed milk.

It's very confusing when we read a chapter like this one, in which we read information that is contradictory to everything we've been taught for the past sixty years. One of the problems is that we often forget about the source of our information. If the only places we hear about saturated fats are government agencies and health organizations, we often won't look to where they are getting their information. Another problem is that if we're told inaccurate or wrong information enough times, we begin to believe it's true. I believe this is what has happened with saturated fats. Once these organizations and government agencies committed themselves to denigrating saturated fats, it's now very difficult to come out and reverse their position on the subject. The reputation and integrity of their statements could be severely tarnished if they were to reverse their position now.

Fat physiology is quite complicated. I've read much on this subject over the last two decades in an attempt to discover the truths about fat in nutrition, health, and disease. I would refer you to my first book on the importance of a balanced fat diet (*42 Days to a New Life*) and to a book by Dr. Mary Enig (one of the foremost fat physiologists in the world), *Eat Fat, Lose Fat*. Another very insightful book about fat physiology and the pitfalls of bad analysis of published data concerning saturated fats and cholesterol is a masterpiece by Dr. Uffe Ravnskov, MD, PhD, *The Cholesterol Myths*. All three of these books review massive amounts of data that contradict government and health organization guidelines.

In February 2015, the Food and Drug Administration released a statement that we no longer need to concern ourselves with the cholesterol content of food, but we still need to reduce saturated fat intake. They stated the reason for the change in this guideline: it "is complicated." The problem with this statement is that most foods that are high in cholesterol are also high in saturated fat. They are found together in most foods (animal, poultry, and fish fats). And as I pointed out earlier, the same portion of Chinook salmon contains the same amount of saturated fat as a similar-sized serving of New York strip steak. You see the conundrum? A three-and-a-half-ounce steak and the same-sized piece of salmon each contain about three grams of saturated fat. Yet we're told that salmon is heart healthy but that steak will cause heart disease and cancer.

While my goal hasn't been to make you into a chemist or an expert in saturated fats, I believe we need to have enough knowledge about them so we don't fear eating them. These fats not only give much flavor to foods we consume but also help our bodies function in many healthy ways. More important is what accompanies those saturated fats. If a chicken was fed cornmeal, as is the case on most commercial chicken farms, or a cow was fed corn silage instead of grass, then you would be eating saturated fats associated with the unnatural corn-induced fat composition of the chicken or the cow (rich in omega-6 fat content) rather than eggs, milk, or meat derived from grass-fed fats (rich in omega-3 fat content). As you learned in previous chapters, excess omega-6 fats lead to inflammation and damage to the body, and higher omega-3 fats lead to healthier cells, immune system, and nervous system. Unopposed inflammation (due to a lack of omega-3 fat) leads directly to heart disease, arthritis, autoimmune disease, osteoporosis, psoriasis, and so forth. See my book *42 Days to a New Life* for a review of these effects on every organ system of our bodies.

Pearls

- Saturated fats are beneficial to our health.
- No association has been found between saturated fat intake and heart disease or stroke.
- The animal's diet is the problem, not its saturated fat content.

CHAPTER 10

Modern Diets:
A Comparative Appraisal

Learn to do common things uncommonly well; we must always keep
in mind that anything that helps fill the dinner pail is valuable.

George Washington Carver

We live in a world with a multitude of choices today. Whether it's
a new automobile, a cell phone, an electronic tablet, television
channels, or a wealth of other items and activities that affect us daily,
we're faced with numerous options. When it comes to diet plans,
we're challenged to select from a wide array of alternatives as well.
When I first began my quest to understand why we've developed so
many medical problems in America, which are now overwhelming the
health care system, I was amazed to realize that our diets are directly
responsible for many of these ailments.

As I proceeded with my research and began educating patients
about the importance of diet choices, they asked me about the best diet
to incorporate in their lives.

Wow! What a loaded question. I had no idea how many diet plans
were available to the American consumer today. Several plans focus
on weight loss, as this is the primary motivator for so many of us

who have put on extra pounds over the years. But there are other diet plans that promote a better way of living in general and better health specifically. Still others focus on a diet plan that promotes a specific belief system, an avoidance of specific foods for various reasons, or a diet that encourages individuals to consume food products developed by individual companies that have a strong motivation for financial gain.

My goal in this chapter isn't to convince you to adopt a specific diet plan. Rather, it's to discuss the pros and cons of several of these diets. I apologize in advance if I failed to cover your favorite diet, but you can always go to my website at http://www.lyonsmedicalnews.com and ask me to review it. I have alphabetized the diets I have chosen to review, since I don't want anyone to think I favor one over another. We all prefer certain foods in our diets. As my chapter on the Lyons Lifestyle will outline, my recommendations can be adapted to many of the various diet plans I discuss.

Atkins Diet

This diet focuses on a weight-loss program that severely limits carbohydrate intake. While the food pyramid the Food and Drug Administration promotes recommended three hundred grams of carbohydrates per day, the Atkins Diet recommends twenty grams of net carbohydrates per day. The diet consists of four phases: induction, ongoing weight loss, pre-maintenance, and lifetime maintenance. Each phase advises specific foods to avoid and/or consume.

The diet is very successful in initiating and maintaining weight loss as long as your compliance is good. It has also been shown to reduce a number of medical problems related to the metabolic syndrome in long-term studies, including high blood pressure and heart disease.

The biggest issues I've heard from patients is that this diet is hard to sustain because of one's constant desire to eat more carbohydrates and the limited dietary options the diet affords to one's palate.

As you advance through the various phases of the Atkins Diet, you're afforded a maintenance plan of seventy-five grams of net carbohydrates per day. As can be seen in my chapter on fructose, this increase in carbohydrate intake could result in activating the metabolic syndrome, since the maximum recommended allowance is ten to fifteen grams of fructose per day. While this may not occur in all of us, care must be taken to make sure you limit your fructose intake.

One concern many people have about the Atkins Diet is that so much protein could potentially harm one's kidneys long term. Data now show that as long as you consume enough saturated fats with your protein, they will protect your kidneys from damage from excess exposure. Additionally, the Atkins Diet doesn't distinguish between protein sources, and recent studies show that protein from soybeans can lead to low testosterone in men, a problem not seen with other sources of protein, such as milk whey protein. While data haven't been produced to explain the reason for this in their findings, soy is rich in omega-6 fatty acids, and these fats have been independently shown to cause this same "low T" effect.

The Atkins Company has developed many products, including drinks and bars that are available in many grocery and pharmacy outlets.

FODMAP Diet

This very specific diet eliminates foods from the diet that can cause gastrointestinal distress. FODMAP is an acronym for "fermentable, oligo-, di-, monosaccharides, and polyols." This diet avoids these sugars and sugar alcohols, since the large intestine (colon) bacteria digest these carbohydrates, producing gas that leads to intestinal distention, bloating, passing gas from the colon, belching, abdominal pain, and altered bowel function. It will also lead to gastric distention and esophageal reflux.

Elimination of FODMAP foods has been shown to dramatically improve these symptoms in affected individuals. The diet is rather restrictive in that you need to eliminate numerous fruits, vegetables, and grains from your diet to be compliant.

Foods high in these sugars include stone fruits (fruits with seeds), wheat, barley, rye, onions, garlic, artichokes, cauliflower, broccoli, brussels sprouts, cabbage, fennel, mushrooms, beans, and chocolate. The stone fruits include apples, apricots, avocados, blackberries, cherries, nectarines, peaches, pears, plums, prunes, and watermelon. Sugar alcohols include arabitol, erythritol, glycerol, hydrogenated starch hydrolysate, isomalt, lactitol, maltitol, mannitol, sorbitol, and xylitol. Our intestinal system digests or only partially digests these, so they are passed into the colon, where bacteria ferment them and generate the gases leading to symptoms.

This diet wasn't designed for weight reduction, but as you can see, if you eliminate this many carbohydrates containing fructose (fruit) and amylopectin (wheat), you may see some weight loss. Regardless, it will have a positive effect on gastrointestinal symptoms and metabolic syndrome if those are problems you're currently suffering from.

Isagenix Diet

This diet plan is a protein-shake-based product that replaces two meals per day with a formulated powder blended into a shake. There are multiple components to this diet plan, including meal replacement whey protein shakes, bars, cleansing products, mineral and vitamin enhancements, natural accelerators, soups, and snacks. The whey protein is derived from New Zealand grass-fed (omega-3) cows. The diet is limiting in that you consume the same shakes day in and day out without a lot of variety. The product will cost about six dollars per day for two meal replacements, but it works because it's a calorically limiting (about 250 calories per breakfast and lunch), high-quality-fat, high-protein formulation that causes you to lose weight in a balanced way as long as you supplement your diet with a source of essential fats (omega-3 and omega-6 fat) somewhere along the way. They provide their own essential fats and vitamin or mineral supplements for this as well. Additionally, vegetarian dietary options are available. The cost can be dramatically reduced or eliminated if you become a multilevel market distributor of the product.

As is true of many of the diet products, it isn't clear from research whether you must stay on this product indefinitely to maintain weight loss. Regardless, the diet works by reducing your caloric intake by about one thousand calories per day and increasing your metabolic rate with a high-protein diet enriched with essential vitamins and minerals. The effects are similar to those seen by the Atkins Diet, but I found no head-to-head diet trials comparing outcomes between Isagenix and the Atkins plans.

Testimonials on their website document results of sustained weight loss, high-energy performance, loss of fatigue, and healthy aging.

Jenny Craig Diet

This is a diet designed to be a nutritionally balanced, weight-reducing plan with coaches who assist you in developing and maintaining the right diet strategy for you. There's no specific restriction on foods, and it works similarly to other diet plans that sell you food. The fundamentals of this diet are caloric restriction, good nutrition, and online or local coaching to help with motivation and insight about your weight and nutritional health.

There's typically a monthly membership fee and the added cost of purchasing their food products. The foods contain animal products, so the plan is rather limiting for vegans or strict vegetarians. The caloric intake is about twelve hundred calories per day. It's also high in protein and low in fat and sodium content. You can supplement their prepackaged foods with fruits and vegetables.

They have extensive exercise, nutrition, and weight coaching as well as online tracking to assist you in staying on course with your weight-loss goals. There's a transition off their foods once you've reached specific goals.

As you've learned, a low-fat intake can lead to several problems. Kidney damage can occur without saturated fats to accompany the protein. Vitamin D deficiency can occur from fat deficiency. I won't repeat the list, but you get the picture. The good part of this diet is the planned discontinuation from the diet before these issues could become relevant.

Mediterranean Diet

This diet is a bit of a misnomer since all diets in the Mediterranean area are clearly not the same. For example, the diet of the people from Northern Italy is quite different from that of Southern Italy. One side of an island in Greece has a completely different diet than the opposite side of that same landmass. A high saturated fat French diet is uniquely different from the rest of the Mediterranean region. Suffice it to say, this popularized diet is advertised as "heart" healthy, but head-to-head studies with an Atkins/South Beach type plan shows that it isn't as healthy as these other two diets in long-term, follow-up studies. Head-to-head trials show, however, that they are healthier for us than the high-carbohydrate, low-fat Western diet we currently consume.

This can be a balanced, unprocessed food diet that includes fresh fruits and vegetables, nuts, fish and seafood, whole grains, beans and legumes, olive oil, low consumption of sweets, meat and meat products, moderate consumption of red wine, and moderate consumption of dairy products and yogurt. One fascinating aspect of olive oil consumption is that prior to World War II, most olive oil was used in the making of soap and lamp oil. This changed during the war when all the farm foods that peasants consumed were used to feed the Italian army. This left the peasants with little else to eat, and they resorted to olive oil as an energy source that helped keep them alive through the war years.

If you consume this diet, you can activate the metabolic syndrome; so you must be careful not to consume excess fruit. True to the Mediterranean Diet, those who don't consume westernized wheat products infrequently suffer from the maladies I mentioned in the chapters on gluten and grains. Good food choices, such as keeping fructose and American grain intake to a minimum on a daily basis, will allow you to safely follow this diet plan. The grain issue is a challenge in America, since many grain products are derived from hybridized and genetically modified cereals.

Nutrisystem Diet

The Nutrisystem Diet is a simplified weight-reduction plan that significantly and simply reduces caloric intake to about one thousand calories per day. It provides three meals and a dessert per day. The diet doesn't discriminate against many foods, only the amount. Over half of the calories are derived from carbohydrates, and the prepackaged food is shipped to your house for quick, convenient consumption. Most of the packages are prepared in the microwave. The meal plan will cost you about ten dollars per day, but you'll certainly lose weight while on the diet to the tune of one to two pounds per week. You're also allowed to supplement the diet plan with fruits and vegetables from the grocery store, but this step only adds more carbohydrates to your diet.

You are advised against using this diet while pregnant or if you suffer from kidney disease, according to the Webmd.com website. As I pointed out in my fructose chapter, excess daily fructose leads to increased uric acid production and could potentially worsen kidney function on a diet that contains so many carbohydrates.

Food options in the Nutrisystem Diet have grown, and this change enables you to be more selective in avoiding excess fructose and other carbohydrates with this diet plan.

Paleo Diet

This recently popularized diet is based on the premise that if the caveman didn't eat it, you shouldn't either. Because of this, you should eliminate all processed foods, dairy products, grains, beans or legumes, refined sugar products, and so forth. The diet consists of meats, fruits, and vegetables similar to an Atkins or South Beach plan. If you can hunt it, fish it, or forage it, then you can eat it. But if it's grown in an orchard or garden, or derived from a food-processing plant, you can't eat it.

Because of the limitations of this diet, many Paleo advocates have modified their interpretation of the diet and include garden vegetables, eggs, and year-round consumption of fruits to provide variety to the palate.

Food choices on your part, while following the Paleo Diet, clearly will dictate your metabolic stability. If you overindulge in fruits and berries, you could activate the metabolic syndrome. Additionally, because the Western diet is omega-3 fat deficient, you would require a supplement such as flaxseed, krill, or fish oil unless you consume plenty of greens, wild game, or fish daily.

SlimFast Diet

This twelve-hundred-calorie diet is easy to follow since the company has developed a product line of snacks and meal replacements. It will predictably lead to about a twenty-pound weight loss, at which time you typically plateau, since this is a high-carbohydrate, high-fiber, low-calorie diet. This plan provides satiety, the feeling of fullness, when you eat a meal, but it won't correct your metabolism if you've activated the metabolic syndrome, since weight will promptly return when you stop dieting.

You should consume one five-hundred-calorie meal, which you prepare for yourself, in addition to using their product line. Their prepackaged foods will cost you about three to five dollars per day if you follow the diet faithfully.

South Beach Diet

A cardiologist developed this diet in an attempt to provide his patients with a meal plan that would lower their risk of heart disease. It's a three-phase diet plan progressing from a very restrictive to less restrictive structure. Although the diet is based on the glycemic index, there are problems with just avoiding foods with a high-glycemic index, since fructose has a low-glycemic index, yet it induces the metabolic syndrome when we consume too much of this sugar on a daily basis.

The diet is based on "good" and "bad" carbohydrates and "good" and "bad" fats, but it basically adheres to the American Heart Association guidelines of avoiding saturated fats. As I pointed out in a previous chapter, the source the saturated fats are derived from is far more important than the saturated fat itself.

People lose weight with the diet since it's low in processed carbohydrates and high in protein, and it avoids trans fats. There's little data to support its claim to reduce heart disease. The primary cost of the diet is the purchase of its manual. There's also an online membership that helps the member with various aspects of dieting and monitoring weight loss, but critics claim that if you consume the foods suggested on a daily basis, your grocery bill will rise. The diet is rich in vegetables, whole grains, eggs, nuts, lean meats, and low-fat dairy products.

Vegan Diet

The vegan diet excludes all animal products, including dairy, honey, beeswax, and eggs. Because of its restrictive menu, you consume fruits, vegetables, grains, nuts, seeds, beans, and legumes. As can be seen from this list, the metabolic syndrome can occur if activated from excess fructose intake from the fruits and grains. If you go through a fructose fast and then prudently add these back to your diet, you can reverse the metabolic syndrome. Just have your metabolic profile checked a couple of times per year to make sure you haven't reactivated it.

Most vegans already know this, but we derive our vitamin B12 from animal sources, so you would need to take a supplement for this essential vitamin. Additionally, this diet is low in many fats, so you need to make sure you get adequate sources of omega-3, omega-6, and saturated fats in your food choices to meet those needs.

Vegetarian Diet

This approach to dieting varies from a vegan (no eggs, dairy, honey, or beeswax) to ovo-vegetarian (includes eggs), lacto-vegetarian (includes dairy), lacto-ovo vegetarian (includes eggs and dairy), or semi-vegetarian (includes fish and poultry on occasion) and other variations, depending on religious, political, or ethnic influences.

These diets have included vegetable oils, and they have caused significant excess omega-6 fat consumption with minimal omega-3 fat intake, so individuals have suffered from inflammatory diseases similar to non-vegetarian diets. As dieters have become educated concerning this error in nutrition, they have remedied this by reducing processed food consumption, switching from vegetable to olive oils, supplementing their diets with omega-3 fats, and limiting their fruit intake. Because of this, studies now demonstrate improved health with this approach. As with the vegan diet, you may need a vitamin B-12 supplement as well.

Some individuals who limit themselves to vegetarian diets now consume only non-genetically modified and organic products in an attempt to further improve their nutrition. While this diet is very sound, it can be rather expensive. As our culture demands better food choices, I believe we will see improvement in this area as well.

Weight Watchers Diet

If you're good at counting points, this diet has proved to be very successful in studies. People lose weight and maintain that reduction if they don't return to their previous lifestyles. This diet allows you to eat any food of your choosing. It works by allowing you to consume a specified amount and kind of food assigned to a point system. You are then allowed to eat food that adds up to so many points per day. Any foods are allowed, so if you have metabolic syndrome in play, you'll need to take specific steps to reverse its effects, as I mentioned earlier.

There's a monthly payment (about eighteen dollars per month) involved with participation with this diet plan, and there are online or local meetings to provide individualized support. The upside is that you can still eat your favorite foods and beverages, just less of them. Weight Watchers carries a limited food line, which will add about thirty dollars per month, and they also have cookbooks you can purchase. As long as you stay on their point system, you will lose weight and maintain it.

As can be seen from this approach, there's no restriction on the type of dieter you are. If you are a vegan or vegetarian, or have another dietary restriction, this diet can still be applied to your preferences.

Zone Diet

This diet was developed as a low-calorie, nutritionally balanced approach that is a low-fat, high-carbohydrate plan. The diet, like most other low-calorie plans, instructs a woman to consume about twelve hundred calories per day and men about fifteen hundred calories per day.

The diet promotes a product line that costs about ten dollars per day and encourages the consumption of fruits and vegetables. If you've activated the metabolic syndrome, this diet will not turn it off if you follow it strictly, since it's too rich in daily fructose intake. Regardless, the diet will lead to and maintain weight loss.

Summary

After reviewing this variety of diets, there are some observations I've made that may be helpful to you. First, many of us struggle with our diets for a variety of reasons. We suffer from excess weight, real or perceived, since some aren't significantly overweight but feel they are. Others of us feel physically, mentally, or spiritually bad with what we eat. Whether we develop gastrointestinal problems from the foods we consume, get migraine headaches, suffer from joint and muscle pains, feel lethargic, or encounter many other complaints attributable to what we eat, we go on a quest to find foods that allow us to feel better or eliminate our maladies.

Some diets help us with improved symptoms, others help us to lose weight, and some allow us to follow religious, ethnic, or political beliefs. Whatever your specific reason for following a diet, one fact is clear: there is probably one out there just for you.

Second, the diets that are successful, at least temporarily, all have you decrease your caloric intake from where you started to around one thousand to twelve hundred calories per day. What that tells me right away is that we eat too much in the first place. The Food and Drug Administration guidelines on food labels are about 100 percent too high for most of us. Just by lowering the amount of what we eat daily, we will take a step leading to significant weight loss for those of us who are overweight. After a twenty- to thirty-pound loss, we will then reach a plateau. If we then give up the diet and return to our previous lifestyle, our weight will promptly return toward our baseline before the diet was initiated. The question we must then ask ourselves is this: can we quit eating the two thousand to twenty-five hundred calories per day and just reduce our meal size long term? That is a challenge given the way foods are packaged and the manner in which restaurants provide larger and larger meal sizes. In the past we ate to live. Now we live to eat. And if marijuana is legalized nationally, food consumption will probably rise further, since smoking pot stimulates the appetite and gives the munchies while reducing brain-induced inhibitions to control food consumption.

Third; consuming many of the diets, especially those that maintain a high carbohydrate intake, won't correct the metabolic syndrome in many of us. You will see an improvement in some areas of your metabolism just because you lose weight, but if you don't go through a carbohydrate fast for a few weeks to shut down the metabolic pathway that has been turned on by daily, excess fructose intake, the metabolic syndrome will often persist during and after the diet.

Finally, some diets are designed to have you support a cause or company's nutritional beliefs and can cost you a lot of money over time. It is important to realize though people consume fast food several times per week and it costs more than many of these diet plans, are not as nutritious and provide too many calories per meal. Regardless of the diet you choose for yourself, employ the guidelines I outline in my chapter on the Lyons Lifestyle. It will work better for you in the long run.

Pearls

- We consume too many calories on a daily basis.
- Numerous diets have been developed to accommodate the many reasons we diet the way we choose.
- There's a diet plan that's most likely right for you.

CHAPTER 11

The New Food Label: An Improvement?

There is nothing so strong or safe in an
emergency of life as the simple truth.
Charles Dickens

If you were to purchase a new car after driving the last one for over a decade, you would assume that the new model you acquire will have dramatically advanced features, given all the major changes that occurred in that time period. There will be new safety features, improved gasoline mileage (maybe it's even a hybrid, all-electric, or hydrogen-fueled model), advanced electronic gadgetry galore, and better design features to meet a multitude of modern consumer demands.

In the food industry, similarly one might also assume that the new food label, which was to be released in 2015 (though this hasn't occurred as of this writing), would be a genuine update to inform consumers of the information relevant to the newest insights in nutrition. This is the first major revision of the nutrient and ingredient content requirement found on most foods we purchase from grocery markets since the US Food and Drug Administration first released it twenty years ago. I wrote a line-by-line analysis of that food label in my second book, *Fructose Exposed*, so I won't rewrite that chapter here. What's important to know about the proposed food label is that some of the most important details we need to know about the contents of what we purchase and consume are either absent or untrue.

First, and most importantly, the food label tells us that if a "serving size" contains less than five hundred milligrams of trans fat per serving, it can be labeled, "Zero grams trans fat" per serving. By manipulating the "serving size," the manufacturer can get a "zero" on the food label very easily. You're still forced to carry your magnifying glass to read the ingredient section to see whether it contains either hydrogenated or partially hydrogenated fats (trans fats) in the myriad of listed ingredients.

Second, the present food label doesn't inform you of the quantity of fructose contained in the package or the serving size. Since over seventy million of us suffer from the metabolic syndrome caused by daily, excess fructose intake, it would be very helpful to have that information at our fingertips when we go shopping. Chapter 9 of my book *Fructose Exposed* contains twenty data tables of many foods found in the grocery store, but most of us don't take the book shopping with us (though, I must say, I have seen shoppers using it at the supermarket where I shop). It's also important to realize that the fresh fruit section of the supermarket has no food label, yet it's there where you'll find some of the highest quantities of fructose in the entire store.

Third, the outdated food label doesn't allow us to know whether omega-3 or omega-6 fats are present or in what quantity. As I pointed out in this and my first book, *42 Days to a New Life*, we consume a massive amount of omega-6 fat, primarily in vegetable oils. We consume almost no omega-3 fats unless we supplement our diets. But there are good sources of omega-3 fat in foods in the store available to you; you must discover these for yourself without the benefit of the food label. The FDA currently lumps omega-3 and omega-6 fatty acids under a general heading of "polyunsaturated" fat. While these are essential fats, you can see that the amount of each of these oils is what is truly important when you're trying to figure out whether you want to consume that product.

Fourth, when we read the food label, the numbers present are based on a fine print "Daily Values" section, which most of us never read. The percentages of all the numbers listed are based on a two-thousand-calorie diet. Most of us get fat on two thousand calories per day, unless we're very active people. The youth of America either aren't active enough or are consuming even more than two thousand calories per day, since millions of children and adolescents are overweight or obese. Regardless, we need to cut the numbers in half, and we want to shoot more toward a one-thousand-calorie diet if we want to avoid becoming obese.

Fifth, the origin of the food that contains saturated fats isn't included in the food label. Why is that important? As I pointed out in my chapter on saturated fats and in my first book, *42 Days to a New Life*, saturated fat per se isn't the important piece of information we need to know when deciding whether we want to eat a specific food. Rather, we need to know what the cow or chicken was fed to know whether its food product is loaded with omega-3 or omega-6 fat. A corn-fed cow will have inflammatory, omega-6 fat with its saturated fats, while a grass-fed cow will have anti-inflammatory, omega-3 fat with its saturated fats. The same is true for chickens and eggs.

Sixth, the presence of "natural" trans fats, also known as conjugated linoleic acid (CLA), is lumped with the "manufactured" trans fats (hydrogenated and partially hydrogenated vegetable oils) on the food label. The FDA allows no distinction, and we, the consumer, don't know the difference. The one thing helpful for you to know is that if an unprocessed meat product contains trans fat on the food label, the label indirectly informs you that this is "natural" trans fat. The reason for this is that "natural" trans fat, or CLA, is found only in grass-fed, not corn-fed ruminant, animals such as cows. The bacterial flora found in these cows' stomachs ferment the grasses they eat, and this fermentation produces the CLAs. When the cows' diet is changed to corn and soybean meal (the predominant diet of feedlot cattle), the bacteria that produce the CLAs die, so the production of CLA stops. The "natural" trans fats (CLAs) have been found to reduce the risk of heart disease, cancer, and obesity; just the opposite is true for "manufactured" trans fats (see the chapter on trans fats). This is a very important distinction we should consider.

This brings us to the new food label. The well-studied and published additions to our knowledge concerning modern nutrition should be defined in the new label. It would stand to reason that if we're trying to reduce our risk of developing the modern diseases plaguing America, we would now be provided with these facts at our fingertips at the supermarket when we examine the next food label. Yet none of these facts have been included. I cannot tell you the reason for this, but if you examine the bibliography of my first two books, as well as the one at the end of this book, you don't need to take my word for it; the science speaks for itself. We all need to know the above-outlined information if we're trying to keep our children and ourselves healthier than what the past sixty years of destructive food consumption have resulted in.

Please review the information I've provided for you so you can make a truly informed decision about what you purchase and consume on a daily basis. Don't rely on the old or new food labels because both are deficient in the six points I outlined above. As you'll see when it's released, the new food label doesn't provide you with any of the important facts I've outlined for you in this chapter.

1. The new food label won't specify how much trans fat is present.
2. The new food label won't inform you about fructose content.
3. The new food label won't let you know whether or how much omega-3 or omega-6 fat is present.
4. The new food label quantities will still be based on a two thousand-calorie (or more) diet.

5. The new food label won't specify the diet of the animals, poultry, and so forth we are consuming.
6. The new food label won't distinguish between natural or manufactured trans fats.

Here are the important considerations when reading food labels:

- Seek out grass-fed animal foods (ask the butcher if it isn't labeled) when possible, since they are higher in omega-3 fats.
- Reduce your omega-6 fat intake (vegetable oils rich in omega-6 fat include cottonseed, peanut, corn, safflower, soybean, sunflower, and sesame).
- Avoid all hydrogenated or partially hydrogenated oils.
- Assume that half of the sugar carbohydrates are fructose unless the ingredient list doesn't contain sugar, high-fructose corn syrup, honey, agave syrup, or fructose, since the label intentionally tries to confuse you on this point.
- Try to keep your sugar-carbohydrate intake less than twenty to thirty grams (ten to fifteen grams of fructose) per day.
- Reduce your total caloric intake to one thousand to fifteen hundred calories per day.
- Finally, you should consider taking a daily multivitamin and a dietary supplement of fish, krill, or flaxseed oil, since omega-3 fats are grossly underrepresented in our Western diet.

Pearls

- The proposed new food label is deficient in adequately informing us about content of trans fats, omega-3 fat, omega-6 fat, fructose, or natural-versus-manufactured trans fats.
- We need to reduce our total caloric intake to about one half of what the food label is currently based on.

CHAPTER 12

What Do Herbivores Do with Carbohydrates?

Of course it's the same old story. Truth usually is the same old story.
Margaret Thatcher

" **B** ut Doctor, fruits are natural! How can you tell me they cause as many problems as high-fructose corn syrup? And, besides, I only eat organic food."

I can't tell you how often I hear this argument when I'm trying to teach patients. Chemistry is pure. Chemistry doesn't care about your political or religious views. It doesn't care about your financial status or ethnicity. Chemistry is a pure science: water is water, no matter where it's found. Carbon dioxide is the same, whether it's the waste product of burning diesel or air I expel from my lungs. Likewise, fructose is fructose. The source doesn't matter. It can come from watermelon or soda pop; it can be found in honey or a fruit smoothie; it's present in a cupcake or an apple. It's all the same, regardless of the source. It's a simple sugar that is metabolized in the human body in a very specific way.

This fact got me to question why so many species of the animal kingdom are herbivores yet live healthy lives. That is, their sole survival depends on the consumption of fruits, grains, grasses, and vegetables.

What happens to those plants in their digestive tracts that allow them to extract enough nutrients without suffering the health issues we now face since we became a high carbohydrate-consuming nation? This question started me on a fascinating and insightful journey that brought me much insight into part of the reason why carbohydrates create so many problems in our digestive tracts.

Some visible examples of carbohydrate metabolism are all around us, but we don't really think about them as they relate to our gut, metabolism, and health in general. For example, we know that if we harvest some grapes and ferment them, we end up with wine. Likewise, if we ferment cabbage, the end product is kimchi. As I researched the digestive systems of herbivores, I learned that there are basically three types of intestines and digestive systems in this portion of the animal kingdom.

These digestive systems include the following:

1. Four-chamber ruminant stomach (cow, goat, sheep, deer, and so forth)
2. Three-chamber pseudo-ruminant stomach (camel and hippopotamus)
3. A functional cecum (rabbit and guinea pig)

What's fascinating about these digestive systems is that they all have one thing in common. All three are modified fermentation vats. While there is anatomic variation among them, each intestinal system processes carbohydrates through a fermentation process provided by a variety of bacteria, yeast, and protozoa. The products of fermentation depend on the carbohydrate consumed and the gut flora present. Just as different kinds of wine depend on the varieties of the yeast and the type of grape being fermented, herbivores produce different digestive end products of fermentation depending on the microbial organisms present in their digestive tracts and the types of carbohydrates they consume.

The important learning lesson here is that *carbohydrates herbivores ingest aren't absorbed as carbohydrates*, as occurs in the human metabolism. *They are the digested and fermented end products of those carbohydrates, which are absorbed into the bloodstream of herbivores.* When cows eat grass, grains, or other carbohydrates, their four-chambered rumen (their version of a stomach) ferments those carbohydrates and converts them into fatty acids, various gases (methane, carbon dioxide, hydrogen, ammonia, and so forth) and other compounds. When a cow chews and ferments the ingested carbohydrates, those foods are passed between the rumen chambers as well as regurgitated into the mouth, where they are chewed again. This process is known as "chewing the cud" (the regurgitated volume of chewed food from partially fermented rumen contents). While the cow chews the cud, up to one hundred liters of saliva are generated and mixed with it each day. This provides water to further the fermentation process when the cow swallows the cud. As a side note, we produce about one liter of saliva per day.

Those compounds that are finally finished with the fermentation process are then passed into the small intestine, where pancreatic and intestinal enzymes and bile further digest them in a fashion similar to the human metabolic process.

Without sounding too crude, I need to explain some basics of digestion that are important for you to know when it comes to understanding how carbohydrates are metabolized. The human colon doesn't absorb nutrients in any meaningful way. The colon ferments foods that haven't been digested in the small intestine with the aid of bacteria, bile, and pancreatic juices. Our digested foods get absorbed from the small intestine and are transported to the liver for further processing. It is the unabsorbed food products that end up in the colon and get fermented by our colon bacteria. That fermentation process leads to gas production in many instances, especially if carbohydrates make their way into the colon.

The functional cecum, the third type of fermentation vat mentioned above, produces digestive products that have no way of being readily absorbed, since the small intestine is upstream from the colon in these herbivores. Functional cecum-endowed animals process their carbohydrates and produce a liquid stool in the elongated, functional cecum they then eliminate, since their fermentation products cannot be absorbed in the colon. The animal then ingests the liquid feces and absorbs the nutrients found in this fermented material; this is similar to our intestinal digestive process. The second pass leads to the formation of the pellets we see in rabbit feces after nutrients from the fermentation and second-pass digestion have been absorbed. For some animals that get their nutrition from a functional cecum, such as horses, volatile fatty acids from fermentation can be absorbed in adequate quantities. The small intestine can absorb many nutrients (primarily proteins, minerals, fats, simple sugars, and vitamins) in these animals as well, but starchy carbohydrates rapidly traverse this area and are poorly absorbed. Of note, they have very few fructose carbohydrates in their diets, and a large starchy carbohydrate load will cause colic in your horse.

As you probably know, the human intestine doesn't contain a fermentation vat, as described in the above three examples. Our intestinal anatomy mimics that of the dog, cat, and pig. Because of this, our intestinal and pancreatic enzyme systems try to process those sugars in a way that is much different than that of herbivores. The consequence is that *when we consume carbohydrates, our small intestines directly absorb those sugars and release massive amounts directly into our bloodstreams.* This process leads to the development of the metabolic syndrome we now witness in millions of Americans (see previous chapter). Had I been a veterinarian, I would have understood that the common thread of carbohydrate processing in humans is quite different than that of herbivores

Regardless, carbohydrates aren't all the same, and when we consume some of them, they do little to alter our metabolism. An example is lemons and limes. They have almost no sugar in them, so when we flavor foods and beverages with their juices, they don't cause us any problems. Quite the opposite is true if we eat a meal consisting of a bowl of fruit with our bagel, a glass of orange juice, and fat-free yogurt laden with fruit and other sweeteners for breakfast. This diet will lead to a massive uptake of carbohydrates, no measurable fat intake, and minimal protein intake. Welcome to the Western diet.

Likewise, most vegetables contain few humanly digestible sugars, so our digestive systems can extract proteins, fats, vitamins, minerals, and water without also extracting large amounts of sugar. Exceptions are sweet corn, sweet potatoes, sugar beets, and sweet peas.

Some vegetables, such as garlic or broccoli and cauliflower, contain sugars (fructans, stachyose, and raffinose, respectively), which colon bacteria process to generate large amounts of gas in the intestines. When we develop intestinal gas, bloating, flatus, and cramping after consuming a carbohydrate, this is because our intestinal bacteria fermented one of those sugars that arrived in our colon. I think it's fair to say that if we're around a herd of cows, we will be amazed by how frequently they belch and pass that intestinal gas. It's amusing how rarely they complain about the effects of carbohydrates on their intestines.

Yet I hear complaints from patients every day because of the effects of carbohydrates generated in their intestines. I want to tell you about a very interesting lady who came to see me as I was researching and writing this book. She had a long-standing history of chronic diarrhea, gas, bloat, and intestinal pain. She had up to twelve bowel movements per day. Several physicians had exhaustively evaluated her. She had undergone numerous tests, including three colonoscopies, three upper endoscopies, three CT scans, and three sets of stool and blood tests. All tests were normal. The reason for three of everything is that she had seen three gastroenterologists.

I took a dietary history, and it became clear to me that her problem was daily, excess carbohydrate intake. I convinced her to stop eating all carbohydrates for a few days. When she did this, she became constipated. She then began to add carbohydrates back into her diet. When she reached thirty grams of carbohydrates per day, she began to have normal bowel movements, but when she reached eighty grams per day, her diarrhea returned. She has challenged and rechallenged herself with the same results. Because she loves carbohydrates, she has learned to "pick her poison," so to speak. She knows that if she overindulges, she will be visiting the commode.

This type of story is true for millions of people. Some of us cannot tolerate lactose (milk sugar), while others cannot tolerate fructose (fructose malabsorption). Still others suffer the gaseous consequences of garlic, broccoli, cauliflower, and the like, as mentioned above. And the list goes on.

In my years as a gastroenterologist, I have been amazed by how many people have developed a medical problem known as small intestinal bacterial overgrowth or SIBO. Thirty-five years ago, it was a relatively rare problem. In the early years, we thought it was just a motility problem, and patients were treated with short courses of antibiotics to eliminate the bacteria that had colonized the small intestine (it usually doesn't contain many bacteria). Then articles began to appear in the medical literature that revealed that daily, excess fructose ingestion caused SIBO to occur. I now realize that it's an attempt our gut has gone through to develop a fermentation vat for the excess carbohydrates we ingest. Bacteria from the colon migrate into the small intestine and feed off the excess sugars we consume. When we stop consuming fructose and other carbohydrates in excess, the small intestine no longer promotes this bacterial overgrowth in most of us.

One thing that is clear from understanding herbivore physiology is that these animals ferment carbohydrates and survive just fine. When we try to become herbivores, we can also survive, but many of the sugars we consume can cause numerous side effects. Many vegans have learned which foods cause gastrointestinal distress, and they learn to eat around them to prevent this problem. Others just ignore the flatus, belching, and bloating, since they enjoy their vegetarian diet immensely.

I would contend that after growing to understand human physiology, herbivore digestion, and the multiplicity of problems and symptoms that arise from consuming so many carbohydrates, we would all do well to understand what is good for us rather than what just tastes good. The health consequences of wrong choices have led to catastrophic results in America's health, including an explosion of high blood pressure, diabetes, strokes, heart disease, obesity, atrial fibrillation, gout, and so forth. It would serve us well to take a long look at our carbohydrate intake as a nation if we truly want to have meaningful health (care) reform in America. We aren't cows or rabbits, nor are our digestive tracts like theirs. Our deteriorating health from excess carbohydrate consumption over the past sixty years reflects that.

Pearls

- Vegetarian animals have a digestive tract that differs from that of humans.
- Animals process carbohydrates differently than humans do.
- Our accommodation to a high-carbohydrate diet is harmful to our health.

CHAPTER 13

Deconstructing Minimalism in Nutritional Health

Anyone who stops learning is old, whether at twenty
or eighty. Anyone who keeps learning stays young. The
greatest thing in life is to keep your mind young.
Henry Ford

My first two books focused on problems in the nutritional health
of Americans: an imbalance of fat in our diets and fructose
metabolism. Soon after that, I realized that an overlap of cause and
effect began to emerge. Not just one cause could be attributed to an
effect; rather, several factors could lead to a common outcome.

Most of us have been caught in a traffic jam on the interstate. We
often conclude that there must have been an accident that impeded the
normal flow of traffic. Yet on some holidays, the traffic may actually
just be an overabundance of automobiles occupying the freeway. Or
it could be rush hour, and an excessive number of individuals decided
to leave work at the same time on that particular day. Or the weather
hampered the visibility, forcing drivers to slow down. You quickly see
that these and other reasons may be the basis for the traffic jam.

If you have a particular cause you fight for, you may focus on just one set of factors to support your cause. An example might be the group of people who believe vaccinations lead to disease in America. Another belief could be that genetic modification and hybridization of food are the cause of disease in America or the conviction that artificial sweeteners, herbicides, pesticides, or hormonal manipulation are the real causes of diseases in America.

While there's probably some truth to many of these statements, minimalism would have us believe that our particular cause is the only one that really matters. Those who have a minimalist view and support a specific tenet will minimize the importance of other possible problems to amplify their position.

When I wrote my first book on the imbalance of fats that has evolved in our diets, it became clear that this imbalance led to a whole new set of ailments in our health. When I was then challenged to find out the facts about fructose, I saw that its excess in our diets led to another set of medical problems. But an overlap began to emerge between the two sets of problems. For example, trans fats were established in the 1950s as the primary cause of heart disease. Yet fructose metabolism has now been shown to lead to the metabolic syndrome and eventually to heart disease. Likewise, omega-3 fatty acid deficiency increases our risk of developing heart disease. And excess omega-6 fatty acid intake will lead to inflammation and sticky platelets; both of these increase our risk of heart disease.

Minimalists would focus on just one issue and not bring all the known contributors and other possible causes together to help us understand the truth about all the reasons why we develop heart disease. America has become a "sound bite" society, and we try to reduce everything to its simplest cause. This minimal, typically singular, approach can leave us with an incomplete answer when we try to figure out these medical issues.

Heart disease is a great example to explore. Several decades ago, it was reported that the cause of heart disease was the excess consumption of saturated fat and cholesterol in the Western diet. As I pointed out in my first book, there are several populations of people on the planet who live on diets very high in saturated fat and cholesterol and don't suffer from heart disease. Numerous modern papers have now debunked this false premise to my satisfaction, but trans fats have also been reported to cause heart disease. Elimination of trans fats has dramatically reduced heart disease in areas of the world, but it didn't prevent all heart disease. Likewise, when omega-3 fatty acids are added to the diet, we see a significant reduction in heart disease. At the same time, daily excess fructose intake alters our metabolism, and a new set of medical conditions develop (high blood pressure, type 2 diabetes, high triglycerides, reduced HDL cholesterol, and elevated LDL and VLDL cholesterol). These predispose us to developing heart disease.

A minimalist approach states that if we just eliminate trans fats, add omega-3 fatty acids, or reduce our daily fructose intake, we will prevent heart disease. But the truth is that all three are important in preventing a heart attack. Additionally, other factors, which are perhaps just as important as these three, need to be considered. Regular aerobic exercise or the inclusion of all essential vitamins, amino acids, fats, and minerals in our diets contributes to the prevention of heart disease.

Nutritional health isn't of just one cause; it's clearly due to several causes. Our challenge is to become vigilant to discover what those causes are so we can truly improve our nutritional health.

The health care industry often convinces patients to take a medication like a statin in an attempt to reduce their risk of heart disease when they have an elevated "bad" LDL cholesterol level during their annual medical checkup. Rather than investigating the type of LDL cholesterol present (large, foamy, or dense/small), trying to identify the cause of the elevated LDL level, or investigating ways to reduce their LDL naturally, the minimalist approach is to have them start taking medication to treat a symptom or achieve a specific effect on a laboratory test result.

We now know that the large, foamy LDL (which many health care providers don't distinguish or understand) isn't a risk factor for heart disease. I will explain this in more depth in the next chapter. If your lab test was actually more comprehensive and found that your large, foamy LDL was the cause of your LDL elevation, you clearly shouldn't have been placed on the statin medication. Likewise, if you have an increased small, dense LDL level, your physician should have investigated your trans fat, omega-6 fat, and fructose intake, since all these cause an elevation of this small, dense LDL cholesterol. I hope you're starting to get the picture.

Whether we focus on the cause of heart disease, stroke, dementia, cancer, arthritis, autoimmune disease, Parkinson's disease, diabetes, or any other specific disease, all these maladies were very rare one hundred years ago. Yet today we all know someone who has or is suffering from one of these diseases. Something changed in the twentieth century that led to the explosion of these and many other ailments. While it's easy to point a finger at trans fats, pesticides, genetic modification of foods, or omega-3 fatty acid deficiency, and so forth, it's clear that a multitude of factors have contributed to the epidemic of medical problems we see in America today.

Minimalism has prevented us from broadening our understanding of the bigger picture of cause and effect, as it relates to nutritional health. Instead, it has us focus on a specific disease of interest or agenda to stop or correct something (eliminate trans fats, stop vaccinating our youth, remove genetically modified foods, eliminate a specific food dye, become a vegan, eat only organic food, give up gluten, and so forth). The list seems endless.

By now I hope you realize that it isn't just one factor that needs to be corrected to improve your health; this goal requires several changes simultaneously. If you focus on only one correction but continue to neglect the others, you aren't likely to accomplish your goals. It may sound like there is so much to balance that it would be difficult, if not impossible, for most people to get a handle on it. My chapter on the Lyons Lifestyle outlines several of those changes that are needed to help you improve your health. Before I go over those with you, there are more issues I need to cover with you in the next few chapters.

Pearls

- Using a minimalist approach to nutrition may prevent you from improving your nutritional health.
- There are often many nutritional causes for a medical malady to occur. They all need to be addressed simultaneously.

CHAPTER 14

Present Guidelines for Nutrition in America

The doorstep to the temple of wisdom is a
knowledge of our own ignorance.
Benjamin Franklin

When Christopher Columbus traveled across the Atlantic to the
Americas, Ferdinand Magellan circumnavigated the globe, or
the Lewis and Clark expedition traveled across the North American
continent, they all went on uncharted journeys. They recorded their
travels with journals, diaries, drawings, and the like so future voyagers
would be better prepared to make a similar journey.

Prior to the twentieth century, people didn't really concern
themselves with nutrients in their food, vitamin supplements, protein
shakes, or the multitude of nutritional focus points that consume so
much of our time today. They just drank their milk, spread butter on
their homemade bread, ate bacon and eggs, enjoyed roast beef and
potatoes; and occasionally, they were treated to apple pie. If people
were hungry, they ate. They couldn't store food very well, so fruits and
vegetables didn't play much of a part in their diets. Likewise, grains

were unadulterated, and they consumed them only when they baked bread, since most people lived on farms or ate farm foods.

Times have changed dramatically in the past one hundred years, and we moved off the farm. We now go to the bakery and/or grocery store regularly, and we supplement our diets with all kinds of vitamins, minerals, fats, proteins, and carbohydrates. In that same time span, we've seen an explosion of heart disease, strokes, cancers, and inflammatory diseases of a variety that boggle the mind. Why? What happened? As these diseases began to consume our lives, academic nutrition and the federal government's agencies began to research and develop policies that now guide us in our dietary choices. But why did these ailments take center stage in America?

As we've discussed, the first change that occurred to ignite our health meltdown was the introduction of trans fats into the Western diet in the early 1900s. The federal government and academic nutrition promoted the use of these fats in the 1950s on advice that farm fats were causing heart disease. As we now know, farm fats aren't the cause of heart disease, nor are other saturated fats; but the damage has already been done. Now the Food and Drug Administration is considering the removal of trans fats from the Western diet. If and when this will occur isn't known at the time of this writing.

The next guidance the Food and Drug Administration delivered to the American public was that we should begin consuming large quantities of fruits, vegetables, grains, and cereals. This was in concert with governmental recommendations that we lower our cholesterol and saturated fat intake and replace those fats with vegetable oils (omega-6) and low-fat food products. Following these recommendations has directly led to the epidemics of heart disease, stroke, kidney disease, high blood pressure, diabetes, cancer, vitamin D deficiency, gallbladder disease, and a multitude of inflammatory diseases affecting virtually every organ system found in our bodies.

In spite of mountains of scientific studies that contradict these guidelines, the federal government continues to promote the same nutritional instruction. First, the Food and Drug Administration, in concert with the Department of Agriculture, began promoting the food pyramid and then the MyPlate nutritional guidelines in an attempt to improve America's nutritional state. Both of these advisory tools recommended the consumption of massive quantities of carbohydrates in the form of fruits, grains, and cereals.

Now we've begun to take over feeding our children. In 2010 the federal government initiated the Healthy, Hunger-Free Kids Act to save our kids from bad nutrition. Part of this law was the implementation of a national school meal program, which provides meals to feed students in kindergarten through twelfth grade. By 2012 this program provided "nutritional" support to thirty-one million youth. The tragedy of this program is that the federal government mandates that meals must be nutritionally balanced, low-cost, or free lunches that must meet meal standards based on "Dietary Guidelines for Americans," which originate with the MyPlate mentioned above.

These dietary guidelines recommend the following:

1. Increase fruit intake (high in fructose and other carbohydrates).
2. Increase vegetable intake (this is good for the most part).
3. Increase whole grain intake (high in carbohydrates).
4. Limit calorie intake (good advice).
5. Decrease sodium intake (bad scientific guidance).
6. Decrease saturated fat and trans fat intake (should be only for trans fats).
7. Decrease refined grain and added sugar intake (good advice).
8. Increase fat-free or low-fat dairy products (causes vitamin D deficiency).
9. Increase seafood intake (bad if deep fried).

While these suggestions might make sense in a country where people are rapidly becoming obese, the science contradicts all but numbers four, part of six, and part of seven. Seafood contains omega-3 fatty acids and is clearly beneficial to our health, as I outlined in a previous chapter. But if you deep fry fish rather than grill or barbecue it, you have now subjected yourself to fish and chips loaded with excessive omega-6 (inflammatory) oils. This is precisely what gets served to our students. Regarding number four, most of us routinely consume too many calories, but we wouldn't feel so hungry if we ate high-quality fats and proteins, and avoided carbohydrates. Number two is problematic because many vegetables, especially greens, are good for us, because of vitamins, minerals, omega-3 fat, and phytochemicals routinely found in these foods. The problem with other vegetables is that some contain quite a large amount of fructose (sweet potatoes, sweet corn, sugar beets, and sweet peas) and other sugars (starches from grains, potatoes, and rice). If consumed in excess, they lead to medical problems.

Low-fat foods reduce our absorption of calcium and fat-soluble vitamins; osteoporosis and vitamin D deficiency (see next chapter) now afflict us by the millions. The vast majority of us need to wear glasses or contacts to normalize our vision due to omega-3 fat and vitamin A deficiency. No one truly knows how many women cannot become pregnant and why the majority of men, by and far, are becoming testosterone deficient because of this guideline.

Salt restriction has become a nightmare as well. The present guidelines advise us to reduce sodium intake, while the science performed over the past seventy years contradicts its reduction to reduce heart disease. People who have followed these recommendations have seen increased death rates compared to control patients who didn't reduce their salt intake. These data have been reproduced over and over again, yet the guidelines haven't changed.

Avoidance of all trans fats, refined grains, and added sugar is truly good advice. The problem is that when we've been told to eat trans fats and now are told not to, when we're told to eat whole grains but not refined grains, and when we're told to consume large amounts of sugars from fruit but not added sugar, we're now so confused about what we should eat and what we shouldn't that I think many of us just give up trying to follow any advice and eat whatever tastes good at the moment.

On Friday, February 13, 2015, the guidance to reduce our cholesterol intake was reversed. For over fifty years, we had been instructed to eat alternative foods and forego or dramatically reduce the ingestion of eggs, butter, cheeses, red meats, and other foods rich in cholesterol. We were to substitute trans fats, vegetable oils, low-fat foods, and lean meats in their place. When the announcement came that cholesterol was no longer an issue in our diets, we were told that it "was complicated," and the media reported nothing further.

The obvious question is this: why is this guidance and these policies put in place if they contradict the medical literature? Furthermore, why are we given such guidance and policies, only to have them changed or rescinded? I'm sorry to say that I must also revert to the FDA's "It's complicated" stance. Decisions involve government, politics, business, and competing interests. This issue is beyond the purview of this work but could easily be the subject of its own book.

The medical literature makes it clear that consuming cholesterol has no effect on our health. The problem with our newfound guideline is that we're still advised to avoid saturated fats with vigor. But any nutritionist will tell you that almost all foods that are rich in cholesterol are also rich in saturated fat. They travel together in the same culinary delights, and it's nearly impossible to follow a "no restriction" of cholesterol and a "continued restriction" of saturated fats diet. An example would be eggs. They are rich in cholesterol and saturated fat, yet all studies reveal that eggs aren't associated with heart disease or stroke. So why do we get the paradoxical advice? If it's okay to eat an egg, which is high in cholesterol, but not okay to eat it because it's high in saturated fat, how do we make sense of this? Hopefully, my previous chapters have helped you understand why this guidance isn't valid.

I'm convinced that after studying thousands of journal articles and reading dozens of books about this very complex subject, the average layperson isn't going to be able to wade through the morass and make sense of all the information. Worse, government agencies and academic/ health organizations provide us with guidance that contradicts the science. My goal in writing this book has been to try to help sort out much of the confusion and provide you with a simple set of guidelines to improve your nutritional health; then this is a tool you can use to implement effective habits in your life.

Most of us are like Columbus, Magellan, and Lewis and Clark when it comes to exploring our nutritional health. I hope to help you navigate your path to dietary choices that help you maintain health, reduce disease risk, and potentially reverse medical conditions that already afflict you because of past nutritional choices.

Pearls

- Many American nutritional guidelines are deeply flawed and contradict medical science.
- If vigorously followed, these guidelines lead to failed nutritional health.
- You can make effective nutritional choices to counteract these flaws.

CHAPTER 15

Vitamin D Deficiency: What Went Wrong?

Learning never exhausts the mind.

Leonardo da Vinci

Centuries ago, when people went to sea for long periods, many died from scurvy. It took time before they realized they needed vitamin C sources in their diets, even though they didn't know what this vitamin was or where it came from. Initially, sailors suffering from scurvy became fatigued. As vitamin C deficiency progressed, their teeth would loosen and fall out; their gums would begin to ooze blood; they would develop bruising under the skin; their skin would turn yellow and pale; they would progress to a loss of sensation in their hands and feet; they would develop wounds that don't heal; and in a matter of weeks, without this essential vitamin, they would die from multi-organ bleeding. Fortunately, we rarely see vitamin C deficiency in this country. In the past, we consumed vitamin C in unpasteurized milk. After the mandate of pasteurization of all commercially processed milk in this country in the 1960s, the Food and Drug Administration promoted the consumption of fresh fruit and vegetables as a way to replace vitamin C in our diets.

Why do I give you this graphic introduction? If a large number of Americans suffered from scurvy, this problem would get our attention and that of the Food and Drug Administration in a hurry. People would die daily. A solution to the problem would be quickly clarified, and our health could be rapidly restored. You see, without treatment, vitamin C deficiency kills us in only six to eight weeks. Vitamin D deficiency is a much more insidious problem and one that is much larger than most of us know, as I will explain.

Vitamin D is an essential vitamin with a very complex biology. I won't try to make you an expert in understanding its chemistry, but what I want you to understand by the end of this chapter is that we're suffering from a man-made problem induced by the same dietary guidelines we discussed in the last chapter. This has led to enormous health consequences.

This vitamin is actually a family of fat-soluble compounds derived from cholesterol metabolism. Sunlight or diet converts cholesterol to these vitamin D compounds and finally into vitamin D's active form in humans with the help of the liver and kidneys.

This essential vitamin is found in oily fish species (such as swordfish, salmon, tuna, sardines, sole, flounder, and mackerel), egg yolks, fish liver oils, beef liver, pork (especially the fatty cuts), chicken (the fatty cuts), turkey (the fatty cuts), beef (the fatty cuts), vitamin-D-fortified milk, ricotta cheese, mushrooms, and alfalfa grass. An inactive form of vitamin D is found in many of these foods, and the body's metabolism activates it through sun exposure, the liver, and the kidneys, as needed. The body can readily absorb this inactive form as long as it's consumed with fat, since vitamin D is a fat-soluble vitamin. As the food list implies, if you're consuming a low-fat diet, you cannot get enough vitamin D absorbed into your body. The consequence will be vitamin D deficiency.

The American people as a whole are now deficient of this essential vitamin. You will often read that it's due to a lack of sunshine for those of us who live in the northern latitudes of America. Yet when the data have been analyzed, about 30 percent in the northern states and 25 to 40 percent of those living in the southern states are vitamin D deficient in healthy individuals. In patients suffering from various diseases, the prevalence of vitamin D deficiency is seen in up to 96 percent of those Americans.

What does this vitamin do for us? First, its metabolism enhances the absorption of calcium, iron, magnesium, phosphate, and zinc. Second, it plays a major role in bone health, including bone growth in children and bone strength as we age. Third, it plays a vital role in maintaining normal muscle function, immune function, inflammation control, and cell division and differentiation into specific cell types. Nearly every cell in the human body has receptors on its outer membrane that communicate with vitamin D.

If it's so vital to human health, how could millions of Americans now be deficient in this essential vitamin? In the 1960s, we were advised to consume a low-fat diet and to convert to trans fats, vegetable oils, and a high-carbohydrate diet. America complied as a society. Additionally, the nutrition programs of our national school lunch programs, military diets, food assistance programs, meals for the elderly, food stamps for the impoverished, and academic nutrition programs launched an assault on fatty foods. Fatty foods supply us with this much-needed vitamin. Additionally, we need to consume the fat with the vitamin so our bodies can absorb it.

If we drink vitamin D-enriched skim or low-fat milk, very little of that vitamin gets absorbed. If we don't eat fatty meats or eggs, we don't get any vitamin D absorbed in that boneless, skinless chicken breast or that 99 percent fat-free ham or turkey breast. The fat and the vitamin D travel together for a reason. *Vitamin D is a fat-soluble vitamin.*

Its solubility in fat is primarily with saturated fats, and this is enhanced by omega-3 fats we don't generally get enough of. Worse, omega-6 fat decreases its absorption, and unfortunately, we get too much of this fat in our diets. As I pointed out in previous chapters, this is the exact dilemma that has arisen from following the guidelines of the Food and Drug Administration.

Several diseases are now associated with vitamin D deficiency. The association doesn't necessarily prove that it's the cause, as we will see. The list of associated diseases and vitamin D deficiency includes the following:

- Obesity
- Metabolic syndrome
- Coronary artery disease
- Depression
- Autism
- Schizophrenia
- Type 2 diabetes
- Atrial fibrillation
- Fatty liver disease
- Dementia
- Tuberculosis
- Clostridium difficile colitis
- Multiple sclerosis
- Idiopathic epilepsy
- Urinary tract infections in renal transplant patients
- Urinary tract infections in children
- Breast cancer
- Other cancers
- Atopic dermatitis
- Autoimmune diseases

This is a partial list, and it's the same list of maladies affecting our health I have written about in my previous books. Hundreds of journal articles can be found in the National Library of Medicine about vitamin

D deficiency. I reviewed two hundred such manuscripts and listed some of them in my bibliography, but suffice it to say, the associations between these diseases and vitamin D deficiency are striking.

One of the fortunate things about trying to connect association to causation is that when it comes to a vitamin, intervention is relatively easy. We give half of a group of individuals who have a disease a placebo, and the other half gets the vitamin. If there's a cause, then we should see an effect with treatment. An example of this can be found in the prevention and treatment of rickets, a bowing of the legs from bone softening due to vitamin D deficiency, which has now been clearly shown to have a cause and effect.

An example of an association without benefit of treatment is fatty liver disease (more on this in another chapter). Supplementing individuals who suffer from fatty liver disease and vitamin D deficiency with vitamin D didn't improve the fatty change in the liver or normalize their liver enzymes. Hence, the association isn't a cause and effect. The same is true for breast cancer, type 2 diabetes, heart disease, autoimmune diseases, infectious diseases, dementia, and the list goes on. The bottom line is that while many disease states are associated with vitamin D deficiency, it isn't the cause of these problems. Treatment with vitamin D supplementation doesn't correct the underlying problem associated with its deficiency. It serves as a biomarker for a bigger nutritional problem, not the problem itself. The solution is to correct that problem, and the vitamin D levels will improve. One previously stated example of this is omega-3 fatty acid supplementation. This fat increases the activated form of vitamin D in our bodies. Most of us have been omega-3 fat deficient since the 1960s. This author is trying to reverse that.

Additionally, we need to consume our vitamin D with saturated fats so they can be absorbed in the first place. We also need to eliminate trans fats and reduce our vegetable oils, which interfere with vitamin D absorption. Just trying to correct a laboratory value (a low vitamin

D level) found in a blood test is minimalistic thinking. We need to implement several dietary changes to correct the cause of this deficiency and hopefully prevent or reverse the associated diseases of vitamin D deficiency.

Pearls

- Vitamin D deficiency is currently present in millions of Americans.
- Saturated fats and omega-3 fats enhance vitamin D absorption.
- Vegetable oils (omega-6 fats) and trans fats block the absorption of vitamin D.
- Vitamin D is a biomarker, not the cause of most of the associated diseases associated with its deficiency.

CHAPTER 16

Gastroesophageal Reflux:
What Matters?

Ignorance is the curse of God; knowledge is
the wing wherewith we fly to heaven.
William Shakespeare

When I was a student in medical school, a medication the Food and Drug Administration approved was released into the American economy that would change Wall Street and the health care industry for the next generation. In less than a year, it became the number one prescribed medication in the United States and was the predecessor to a string of medications that have dominated the pharmaceutical landscape, health insurance plans, and now entire shopping aisles of your favorite grocery store ever since. Tagamet, a medication that reduces acid production in the stomach, became the first "blockbuster" medication to ever be produced when its sales surpassed $1 billion a year in worldwide sales for the first time in pharmaceutical history.

Over the next three decades, an army of similar medications were developed and released. They joined Tagamet as the next "blockbuster," and you've heard many of these brand names: Zantac, Pepcid, Axid, Prilosec, Prevacid, Protonix, Aciphex, Nexium, and other look-alike medications that followed. These medications have been prescribed to hundreds of millions of people in the world over that time span. Why?

That question takes me to the subject of this chapter: gastroesophageal reflux disease (GERD). This is a problem of regurgitating gastrointestinal contents from the stomach into the esophagus (our swallowing tube), which leads to a myriad of symptoms and complications. Nearly one-third of us now suffer from GERD on a regular basis; this has led to the explosion of the prescribed (and now over-the-counter) medications I outlined above. How did so many people quickly develop GERD? The first published case of esophageal cancer related to GERD was only in 1954. This has been the fastest-growing cancer in the United States over the past forty years. Liver cancer is now overtaking it, and I will cover this issue in the next chapter.

In preparation for writing this chapter, I visited the Mayo Clinic, WebMD, and National Institutes of Medicine GERD-related websites. They all stated the same dogma: GERD occurs more frequently for those who are pregnant, those who are obese, those taking certain medications and foods, smokers, and the like. I have attended approximately twenty esophagus conferences over the past thirty-five years to keep abreast of the developments related to GERD, and it amazes me that what I will cover in this chapter hasn't been highlighted at any of the conferences or the above-named websites as it relates to taking care of patients whom GERD has often incapacitated.

Several years ago, a young woman was referred to me because she had lost her voice. She could speak only in whispers. This condition was devastating to her, since she was a recording artist and had songs frequently heard on music radio stations. A number of specialists had thoroughly evaluated her and concluded that nothing structurally or physiologically was wrong. I evaluated her and found that she was suffering from GERD. She denied having heartburn, chest or abdominal pain, difficulty swallowing, or regurgitation of gastric contents. I found that she had a hiatal hernia and Barrett's esophagus, a precancerous change to the lining of the esophagus that occurs from chronic GERD. I referred her to surgery, where she underwent a hiatal hernia repair. Six months later, she was singing again, and at the one-year anniversary of her surgery, she was recording music again.

Why is this important? All three websites I mentioned above emphasize that people who suffer from GERD complain of heartburn, chest pain, regurgitation, or difficulty swallowing. A colleague of mine—who was an ear, nose, and throat specialist—and I realized many years ago that most men present with these symptoms while most women don't. Women more frequently have chronic cough, hoarseness, or loss of voice, raspy voice, wheezing, ear aches, and the like. Some women note a lump in the throat and even difficulty swallowing, but their symptoms are distinctly different from those of their male counterparts, who suffer from GERD. The reasons for these differences aren't addressed in the medical literature, and I've never heard a lecture discussing the differences. The significance of this distinction is very important: many women will be significantly delayed or won't be diagnosed with GERD because their symptom complex doesn't fit the academic dogma in textbooks and algorithms used to guide practitioners with GERD management.

I had just finished writing the first draft of this book when a patient asked me a simple question: "Why do I get reflux symptoms when I eat carbohydrates? When I don't eat them, I don't have reflux." I found this fact to be profound, since the only time I get heartburn is after consuming carbohydrates, and I just thought I was the weird one. You see, nowhere in the textbooks, algorithms, or websites is there any mention of this association. I decided that I needed to look into this issue further because I know carbohydrate intake has dramatically increased since the 1960s. In that time span, we've increased carbohydrates from 25 percent to 65 percent with the food pyramid and up to 75 percent with the MyPlate guidelines.

When I researched this association—carbohydrate consumption

and worsening esophageal reflux—in the National Library of Medicine, I was surprised, to say the least, by what I found. Several comments are in order. Obesity has dramatically increased in the United States over the past thirty years. Central obesity occurs with the metabolic syndrome, as I pointed out earlier in chapters 5 and 8. This increased pressure in the abdominal cavity from deposition of excess fat is strongly associated with worsening esophageal reflux, and studies show that losing as little as ten pounds of belly fat can dramatically reduce GERD. The cause of metabolic syndrome and central obesity is carbohydrate ingestion. When you dramatically reduce carbohydrates from your diet, belly fat disappears.

We've also been taught that caloric density (high fat intake) is a cause of GERD. Recent, well-performed studies, however, demonstrate that altering fat intake doesn't change the amount of GERD. To the contrary, it's meal volume that is more important than the caloric density of the food we eat. But the real shocker to me was the volume of medical papers that documented GERD symptoms and esophageal damage from the reflux that significantly improves on a low-carbohydrate diet. Additionally, colonic bacterial fermentation of carbohydrates we cannot absorb in the small intestine leads to increased esophageal reflux by all known measurable parameters that document GERD.

While the total reason for relaxation of the sphincter between the esophagus and stomach leading to the reflux isn't totally clear yet, this carbohydrate fermentation in the colon causes excess release of a hormone called glucagon-like peptide 1 (GLP-1), which accounts for part of this phenomenon. There may be other mechanisms as well, and this is an area of active research because of the millions of people plagued by esophageal reflux. Regardless, the GLP-1 causes gastric distention and delayed emptying of our stomachs (gastroparesis) after we've eaten that bowl or two of pasta. As the stomach enlarges, we feel bloated. Additionally, the lower esophageal sphincter is stretched open; this leads to relaxation of the sphincter, and we begin to belch, hiccup, and reflux gastric contents into the esophagus. This phenomenon doesn't occur immediately after your meal. Its onset begins a few hours after your meal. This accounts for much of the reflux that awakens us from sleep, coughing from regurgitated gastric contents that irritate our throats and lungs. I hear this story virtually every day in my clinical practice.

The next thing we need to understand is why so many of us are developing a hiatal hernia. We've seen doubling in the prevalence of hiatal hernias in America in the last four decades; over 50 percent of us have now developed one. I'll try to best exemplify the phenomena of meal volume with carbohydrates using a real-time example.

Think about spaghetti or macaroni noodles for a moment. You boil them on the stove until they are tender; you rinse them to stop the cooking process and then perhaps mix in a bit of olive oil or butter to keep them from sticking to each other. You then add your favorite sauce and cheese, and partake of these delightful dishes, often accompanied with bread sticks or slices flavored with garlic. You dive into the mountain of carbohydrates, sometimes even delighting in a small second helping. After your meal, you begin to feel that somehow that meal gets bigger in your stomach. Now go look in the pan where you cooked the noodles.

If a few still remain with a bit of water, you soon discover that the noodles are five times bigger than those you served. That same swelling that occurred in the pan is happening in your stomach. What's more, some of those carbohydrates are now making their way into your colon, where bacteria begin the fermentation process leading to reflux. We've always blamed the sauce for inducing esophageal reflux, but it doesn't matter to me what I put on my pasta noodles. I suffer from the reflux problem, all the while blaming the sauce. Data I reviewed and mentioned here blame the noodles or carbohydrates.

In my lifetime as a physician, there has been a steady increase in the prevalence of hiatal hernias in the American population from 30 percent to roughly 50 percent today. This is a mechanical tearing of the diaphragm ligaments at the junction between the stomach and esophagus. Think about a balloon for a moment. The more air you place in the balloon, the shorter the neck becomes. This is a good analogy of what occurs when we fill our stomachs with these carbohydrates, which rapidly expand after ingestion, shortening the balloon neck and creating a hiatal hernia. At the same time, seventy million Americans now suffer from metabolic syndrome and perhaps even more with central obesity, caused by carbohydrates, which place even more pressure on the gastroesophageal junction, helping to produce their hiatal hernia.

Another fascinating observation is that patients who suffer from GERD and consume a gluten-free diet are free of GERD in a two-year follow-up study. This statistic is compared with recurring GERD in 85 percent of individuals without celiac disease, who continue to consume gluten in their diets. The question then arises: is this problem due to the gluten or to the avoidance of wheat and other gluten-based carbohydrates?

There are clear associations between the consumption of foods and beverages that relax the gastroesophageal valve, leading to worsening reflux transiently. Peppermint, coffee, tea, cola, and chocolate all cause relaxation of the area between the esophagus and stomach, which will lead to worsening GERD symptoms. Diminishing these substances in the early afternoon allows for the relaxation effect of the sphincter to wane by evening when we go to bed at night. If we've been consuming carbohydrates all day, though, we will continue to be miserable in spite of avoiding these relaxants. Far more important than giving up your morning coffee (which has several proven benefits), it would be far better to give up your bagel, breakfast cereal, pancakes, waffles, toast, or a multitude of other carbohydrates we begin our day with during breakfast. Additionally, we need to keep our fructose intake to a minimum so we don't activate the metabolic syndrome (see previous chapters) and promote central obesity.

The present guidelines for the treatment of GERD include reduction of meal size independently of what we are eating. We're also advised to avoid the above mentioned foods and beverages as well as spicy or citrus foods. We're also instructed to wait two to three hours after eating before we lie down for bed. From there we move into weight loss, over-the-counter and prescribed medications, elevation of the head of the bed (often a slippery slope), avoidance of tight-fitting garments, and finally, a surgical repair of the hiatal hernia as a last resort. While I don't disagree with the guidelines, my perspective is that if we dramatically reduce carbohydrates to the level of consumption seen in the 1950s (about 25 percent of our diets), all the while reducing belly fat, we will witness a dramatic reduction in GERD in the United States.

This isn't currently part of the recommendations in the management of GERD. Additionally, one of the best medications that cuts back on the symptoms of GERD temporarily and nearly instantaneously is alginic acid or sodium alginate. Numerous papers substantiate the benefits of this seaweed extract in the management of GERD, yet none of the websites I visited even mention this therapy. Perhaps it's because it is an over-the-counter, inexpensive remedy that has almost no side effects; it is very poorly absorbed (leading to less potential side effects) and is a generic plant extract. Regardless of the reasons, many patients in my practice are intolerant of nearly all the prescription medications, yet they derive significant benefit from alginic acid.

If you suffer from GERD, I recommend that you seek medical advice, especially since esophageal cancer can develop from long-standing reflux. I would also encourage you to try my approach: I encourage patients to dramatically reduce their carbohydrate intake daily, increase omega-3 fats to promote reduction in inflammation, avoid omega-6 vegetable oils and trans fats (as these induce inflammation and possibly cancer), and take a multivitamin daily to promote the beneficial effects of omega-3 fats (see previous chapters). There's still a place in the management of many individuals who suffer from GERD to be placed on prescription medications or even undergo surgery, but I strongly encourage them to at least try my more conservative approach first. I've seen thousands of compliant patients who've been able to reduce or eliminate their acid-blocker medications. They may still need the occasional GERD rescue with alginic acid after a decadent gastronomic experience, but for a foodie like me, that seems worth it. While this doesn't produce another Wall Street "blockbuster" medication, it does provide you with an alternative to taking more powerful and potentially more toxic medicines to manage your GERD.

If these changes in our diets were implemented naturally, we would witness marked improvement in our GERD-associated symptoms. This would leave more money in our pockets to spend on other things, such as better-quality food, and at the same time save tens, if not hundreds, of billions of dollars annually in health care expenditures. This is true health care reform.

Pearls

- Carbohydrates worsen hiatal hernia formation and GERD symptoms.
- Carbohydrates cause central obesity, which increases GERD.
- Changing our diets may dramatically reduce GERD in many of us.

CHAPTER 17

Nonalcoholic Fatty Liver Disease: The Newest Epidemic

It may be hard for an egg to turn into a bird: it would be a jolly sight harder for it to learn to fly while remaining an egg. We are like eggs at present. And you cannot go on indefinitely being just an ordinary, decent egg. We must be hatched or go bad.

C. S. Lewis

If you were to take a trip to your local mall and began noticing that every tenth child and every fourth adult had three arms, you might have a rather dramatic reaction. You might ask how this defect could affect so many people at the same time. You could conclude that a drug might be causing this "birth defect," or you might arrive at another plausible answer to explain the phenomenon you're witnessing. When an abnormality is outwardly obvious, we take note immediately, but if the abnormality takes place inside our bodies, no one can notice. Such is the case with nonalcoholic fatty liver disease.

This type of liver damage (we will abbreviate it as NAFLD) is now the most widespread liver disease in adults and children alike, and it's now damaging people's livers across the globe. While alcohol and viral hepatitis can damage the liver, NAFLD causes liver injury in 600 percent more people than alcohol and even more with viral hepatitis. Why? What has led to this new epidemic?

While there are many causes of NAFLD (most are rare or nearly nonexistent), over 90 percent of individuals with NAFLD suffer from metabolic syndrome (see chapter 5). Obese individuals have fatty liver 84 to 96 percent of the time, and insulin resistance is associated with 75 percent of those afflicted with NAFLD. We assume we must be fat to have fatty liver, but 29 percent of NAFLD patients are lean. As we learned from chapter 5, lean people also suffer from metabolic syndrome due to their excess consumption of fructose.

What's even more shocking is that NAFLD wasn't a recognized problem in the United States until the 1980s; now it has reached epidemic proportions. The clues as to why this is so have been discussed in earlier chapters, but I believe we need to realize that NAFLD affects more and more individuals each year and that it won't be reversed until we know it's present and then change our diets so we can reverse the damage smoldering in our livers.

As you can see from the strong associations with obesity, metabolic syndrome, and insulin resistance (type 2 diabetes), the light is probably coming on for you. This clustering of medical problems keeps surfacing with many problems I have been trying to highlight in this book. Suffice it to say, they are all related because they are all caused by the same problem: our Western diet of low-fat, high-carbohydrate, trans- and omega-6-fat-laden foods and excess fructose.

I first became aware of this connection, and I reversed most patients' fatty liver damage when I could get them to start supplementing their diets with omega-3 fatty acids (fish, flax, or krill) and could stop their trans fat intake. This step worked in most individuals, but there was still a subset of patients who didn't get better. When I figured out the fructose connection to fat deposition in the liver through metabolic syndrome, I began having patients fast from fructose if they continued on with progression of their fatty liver disease. Lo and behold, the rest of the patients began to normalize their liver chemistries, their diabetes improved, and their central obesity began to melt away if they remained compliant to my guidelines. I must say, though, that fasting from carbohydrates for three weeks is a hurdle many find nearly impossible to overcome when their metabolism has become addicted to the effects of fructose and grain carbohydrates over decades of excess intake.

Why is it important to control NAFLD? If the disease process is allowed to progress, one can develop cirrhosis of the liver. This, in turn, leads to liver failure and cancer. What's worse, if you suffer from hepatitis C, are a smoker or a pot smoker, or abuse alcohol in addition to having NAFLD, you most likely will arrive at end-stage liver disease much more quickly than if you don't fit into one of these groups. We now have millions of Americans who are infected with the hepatitis C virus; even more smoke tobacco and/or marijuana and/or drink alcohol regularly. In other words, we're growing a third arm—and very rapidly.

What can be done? First, you need to find out whether you're suffering from NAFLD. This requires a blood test and an ultrasound of the liver as a minimum. You may also need to undergo a battery of lab tests, and sometimes a liver biopsy is needed to establish the diagnosis. Once you know whether you're one of the 25 percent of afflicted adults in the United States, you need to aggressively implement the guidelines I've developed throughout this book. You need to reverse metabolic syndrome if it's in play, dramatically reduce omega-6 fat in your diet, and eliminate trans fats. You also need to include an omega-3 fat supplement and a multivitamin as well as drastically decrease fructose in your daily diet. Finally, you need to have your physician monitor your liver to make sure you're effectively reversing NAFLD. Make sure that third arm disappears.

Pearls

- Nonalcoholic fatty liver disease now afflicts one-quarter of the adult population in America.
- This is caused by several factors occurring simultaneously: excess omega-6 fats, trans fats, and omega-3 fat deficiency, along with metabolic syndrome induced by daily, excess fructose ingestion.
- Excess grains intake in individuals who have activated metabolic syndrome advances the fatty liver.
- Tobacco, marijuana, and alcohol can accelerate the disease.
- Nonalcoholic fatty liver disease is reversible in most individuals who are willing to implement vigorous dietary changes.

CHAPTER 18

Nutrition and Heart Disease

To be wholly devoted to some intellectual
exercise is to have succeeded in life.
Robert Louis Stevenson

Prior to the twentieth century, no data had been gathered that documented disease frequency in the United States, since the federal government hadn't grown to its present size to accommodate such activities. What's clear from the early textbooks of medicine and autopsy studies Dr. William Osler, the father of modern medicine, performed is that heart disease was almost never seen in the late 1800's. Additionally, numerous diaries, journals, histories, and biographical books didn't reveal any significant heart disease in America. At the same time, we knew much about the causes of epidemics following the discovery of germ theory. Beginning in the 1600s, Anton van Leeuwenhoek observed the first bacteria under a microscope. Various discoveries over the next two hundred years led to the work of Louis Pasteur and Robert Koch in the 1860s, which proved that germs were the cause of these epidemics.

Dr. Osler was one of the founding physicians of Johns Hopkins University. He was the author of the first medical books that documented the natural history of disease processes. He would perform autopsies of patients who had expired and review their entire medical histories over their lifetimes. By marrying the clinical and pathological information, he was the first physician to document how diseases occur in the way we understand them today. We suffer from symptoms (pain, stiffness, nausea, and so forth) related to a disease process. We then seek out a physician who listens to our story by taking a medical history. He or she then looks for signs (swelling, rash, skin change, abnormal lung, or heart sounds with a stethoscope, and so forth) of the disease by performing a physical examination. Your health care provider will then proceed with laboratory, radiological, or other imaging and testing to confirm a diagnosis leading to a specific treatment. Dr. Osler was the master at bringing the medical history together with the symptoms and signs of disease leading to the patient's death. By doing so, he was able to construct the natural history of the disease. As he proceeded to gather data, heart disease was notably absent in the late 1800s and early 1900s when he was vigorously defining the common maladies that caused death in America.

Fast-forward to present-day health care, and we see that the number one cause of death in the United States is heart disease. Stroke and other vascular disease are also major causes of death. All were so rare that they weren't considered a problem in our health during the time of Osler. Something dramatically changed at the end of World War II. Within the matter of a few decades, heart disease went from a nonentity to a major killer. In the 1950s President Dwight Eisenhower suffered from a heart attack, and our focus on heart disease took center stage in America. Major investigations were launched to discover the cause. As I mentioned earlier, we got off track by blaming saturated fats and cholesterol in our diets as the cause. Nina Teicholz wrote a brilliant historical essay on the details leading to the recent exposure to nutritional fraud perpetrated on the American people in her book, *The Big Fat Surprise*. For those interested in understanding all the historical facts that led to the wrong conclusions, I would encourage you to read her masterpiece.

But what about the cause of heart disease if it's not due to the saturated fat and cholesterol found in our diets. As I pointed out in my chapter dealing with minimalism, there isn't just one cause. It's truly multifactorial and a bit complicated. We first learned that certain types of cholesterol are altered in patients who suffer from a heart attack. These include a low level of HDL cholesterol and an elevated level of LDL cholesterol. Because of these associations, we labeled these blood markers as "good" HDL and "bad" LDL cholesterol. What's unfortunate is that association doesn't necessarily define causation. Additionally, as scientific understanding of LDL proceeded, the knowledge wasn't transmitted to health care providers or patients.

We now know that LDL cholesterol can be broken down into two specific types: large, foamy particles; and small, dense particles. The large, foamy ones have no association with heart disease, while the small, dense ones do. In the 1950s, we didn't know this vital information. What scientists did know was that when we consume saturated fats, our LDL cholesterol goes up. The problem is that we now know it was the large, foamy LDL (the harmless type), and the small, dense LDL isn't affected. In the interim, no one has helped us understand this very important distinction, and millions of Americans have been placed on statins at a cost of nearly $30 billion annually in an attempt to lower our LDL cholesterol. We've also seen the evolution of stricter guidelines to lower our saturated fat intake in an attempt to lower our LDL cholesterol. You can see the fallacy of believing a high LDL cholesterol level is bad. We need to know which type of LDL— small, dense; or large, foamy—is elevated.

One marker of heart disease has been the association of low HDL cholesterol in people who suffer from this malady. It has a higher association than elevated LDL cholesterol when it comes to heart disease, but the pharmaceutical industry has been unable to develop a medication that will safely raise our HDL cholesterol, so this fact somehow gets swept under the carpet. What's even more disconcerting is that when we consume saturated fats, our HDL cholesterol goes up. This is exactly what we want to see if we're trying to reduce our risk of heart disease. So let me review: saturated fats raise our "good" HDL cholesterol and raise our large, foamy LDL cholesterol (the cholesterol that has no association with heart disease). It has no effect on our small, dense LDL, which is associated with heart disease. We can now see from the mountains of data kept from the American people and health care providers alike that saturated fats aren't the cause of heart disease and may actually be beneficial in its prevention.

So if saturated fats aren't the problem, what's the cause of heart disease? One of the major changes in the Western diet in the first half of the twentieth century was the introduction of trans fats by Proctor and Gamble. Crisco was the quintessential fat in the beginning, but several other companies were quick to get on the bandwagon after it was determined that farm fats (saturated fats) were the cause of heart disease. But as science and history have demonstrated, these trans fats have now been definitively linked to heart disease. Those in the European Union and other countries have taken major steps to eliminate them from their diets, and they are returning to saturated fats in the production of many processed foods. But while trans fats are a contributor to heart disease, another bad actor entered the nutritional scene in the last half of the century. The introduction of vegetable oils (rich in omega-6 fatty acids) compounded the problem of heart disease, as these oils induce inflammation in the body.

Numerous studies were performed in the 1970s to the present time, in which Americans were placed on a low-fat, high-carbohydrate diet that included vegetable oil. The investigations didn't reduce heart disease in long-term, follow-up analyses, and one of the concerning aspects of these low-saturated-fat and cholesterol-diet interventions was that many saw an increased number of people developing cancers and gallbladder disease. Additionally, we now see an explosion of vitamin D deficiency and an increase in suicides and violent deaths in participants of these studies. Not much comment was made about these findings, and even less was said about the lack of any meaningful reduction of heart disease in these studies.

As diet intervention studies failed miserably in trying to reduce heart disease and statin therapy escalated to tens of billions of dollars per year without major declines in heart-related death, investigators continued to try to solve the conundrum. While data emerged that heart disease is actually worse on a low-fat diet, we still didn't have a clear picture of the causes yet, since another major change occurred as a consequence of leaving a high-fat diet and consuming a high-carbohydrate diet. This latter diet leads directly to metabolic syndrome (see chapter 5). Data are now clear that the best predictor of increased risk for developing heart disease is the presence of metabolic syndrome. Consumption of any type of fat doesn't cause this syndrome. The primary actor here is daily, excess fructose. Throw in massive increases in the consumption of amylopectin from wheat and other grain products, and seventy million Americans now suffer from metabolic syndrome. Additionally, millions of children and adolescents are developing this problem.

Just as we decreased our saturated fat and cholesterol consumption in an attempt to reduce heart disease, we are now vigorously educated to eat a diet that is rich in fruits and grains, since this is supposedly healthy for us. Yet these foods lead directly to metabolic syndrome when consumed in excess, as is presently the case for most of us. The excess sugar found in these commodities overwhelms our metabolisms, and we are programming ourselves to develop heart disease and strokes.

As can be seen, we've followed a path of nutritional decisions, which have led to worsening health. These changes can be summarized as follows:

1. Reduction of saturated fat and cholesterol in our diets
2. Addition of trans fats
3. Addition of vegetable oils (corn, safflower, peanut, soybean, cottonseed, and so forth)
4. Loss of omega-3 fat from the Western diet (corn-fed rather than grass-fed animals)
5. Introduction of excess carbohydrates (fruits, grains, high-fructose corn syrup, and so forth) to replace farm products

While each of these has independently caused a negative effect on our health, as I have previously discussed in specific chapters, all these changes together have led to devastating damage to our bodies, not just with heart disease but with inflammatory diseases of all types. We cannot correct just one of these problems and expect to solve our medical problems; rather, we need to reverse all of them simultaneously. This is a major challenge for most of us, since erroneous information has conditioned us for the past sixty years. I've found it difficult to educate some people about all these points, because they are so conditioned to continue with what they've been eating for the past several decades. I heard a specific individual say on national talk radio, when a major study revealed the damaging effects of marijuana on a specific part of the human brain that he wouldn't care if he suffered brain damage as long as he could smoke marijuana.

So it goes with some individuals who want to continue consuming several servings of fruit daily; enjoy their cinnamon roll with their morning coffee; and delight in pizza, pasta, bread, or other wheat products several times per day. You get the idea. The problem is that chemistry is chemistry when it comes to the human metabolism. The chemical reactions that lead to heart disease occur in the majority of us when we consume the foods that contain the chemical reactions leading to heart disease, inflammatory diseases, and cancer.

The Lyons Lifestyle chapter outlines recommendations we all need to implement as we seek to reverse the damage occurring in our bodies because of the Western diet.

Pearls

- Heart disease and strokes aren't caused by just one problem in our diets.
- Saturated fat and cholesterol in our diets aren't the causes of heart disease, and strokes and some data suggest a degree of protective effects.
- Eliminating trans fats dramatically reduces heart disease.
- Omega-6 fat excess and omega-3 fat deficiency contribute to heart disease.
- Preventing or reversing metabolic syndrome (caused by excess fructose and worsened by grains) dramatically decreases our risk of heart disease and stroke.

CHAPTER 19

Probiotics: Ready for Prime Time?

Each life is made up of mistakes and learning, waiting and
growing, practicing patience and being persistent.
Billy Graham

When we find ourselves in the yogurt aisle of the grocery store and
see labels on several dairy items, labels that promote the use of
probiotics to improve various ailments, and then query their utility in
our own health at the next office visit with our health care provider, a
conundrum arises. Our physician may often make statements such as,
"They won't hurt you" or "They might make you feel better"; or, if they
were dead honest, they might throw in, "I am not sure of their true
benefit." The last statement is probably the most accurate, as I will try
to explain in this chapter.

First, let's try to understand what a probiotic is before we look at
its potential benefits. Probiotics are defined as live bacteria that convey
beneficial effects on us when we consume them in adequate numbers.
While antibiotics destroy or suppress the growth of bacteria and are
used to fight infections, probiotics typically prevent inflammation.

The normal human gut contains over five hundred species of
bacteria, which weigh up to half a pound and outnumber the cells that

comprise our entire bodies by a factor of ten to one, numbering over one hundred trillion bugs. This normal gut flora produces several products that benefit our health and include folic acid, vitamin K, several B vitamins, and short chain fatty acids. Additionally, these bacteria help process the fiber found in fruits, grains, and vegetables that would otherwise pass through our colons without digestion or fermentation. The products of this fiber and carbohydrate digestion are the formation of a bulky stool, intestinal gas, and facilitation of a bowel movement without constipation or diarrhea.

Diet, antibiotics, and infections can alter the normal gut flora. This change can lead to inflammatory reactions in the intestine as well as affect us systemically. Probiotics are then consumed in various preparations in an attempt to either reduce that inflammation or reorganize the gut flora so it provides long-term symptom relief from the inflammation the initial insult induced. Likewise, some bacteria that infect our intestinal tract can cause diseases to develop. One well-studied infection of the stomach is *Helicobacter pylori*. An infection from these bacteria causes chronic gastritis, peptic ulcers, gastric cancer, and intestinal lymphoma in the susceptible host. It can also lead to chronic anemia and irritable bowel syndrome. Eradication of this infection using antibiotics with supplemental probiotics improves eradication rates and reduces side effects associated with the treatment of the infection. Effective treatment of this bacterial infection reverses the risks of developing the above mentioned diseases in many circumstances.

While we can quickly restore our intestinal flora after antibiotic use or recovery from an infection, when we add probiotics to our daily intake for the next couple of weeks, we can also potentially prevent secondary infections from occurring. Examples of this would be yeast infections and Clostridium difficile infection. Existing data suggest the benefits of probiotics, but they aren't ready for prime time, since there is no consensus yet as to which probiotics should be used. To the contrary, the American Academy of Pediatrics now recognizes the benefits of treating children with antibiotic-associated diarrhea and infectious diarrhea with probiotics. Three different strains of *Lactobacillus* and *Saccharomyces boulardii* probiotic bacteria have been found to be effective in reducing symptoms in these settings. The conclusion? I believe we will have more data, and consensus will eventually be reached, but we aren't there yet for adult intervention, while pediatric consensus has been reached.

Our diets can also alter the gut flora as long as we continue to feed our intestinal bacteria food, which led to their alteration. That alteration may now predispose us to develop an irritable bowel, type 2 diabetes, or migraine headaches and the many other studied diseases that have been reported in the medical literature. The dietary impact of consuming trans fats, vegetable oils (excess omega-6 fat), and excess sugar-containing carbohydrates has immense impact on the gut flora. For example, if we consume excess sugar-containing carbohydrates daily for weeks on end, we can cause bacteria to colonize the small intestine. This bacterial colonization is known as small intestinal bacterial overgrowth or SIBO. SIBO causes significant intestinal distress in many people, since the bacteria produce intestinal gas and partial maldigestion. Probiotics can improve symptoms in this scenario, since these newly introduced bacteria compete with the SIBO bacteria in an attempt to normalize the gut flora.

At this juncture, it isn't well understood how much impact we can have in reversing an abnormal gut biome, caused by dietary influences from consuming excess sugars, trans fats, or omega-6 fats; but we do know they are culpable of altering the bacterial species and numbers of bacteria, and inducing chronic medical problems, such as a leaky gut. In this situation, even though you consume probiotics for these problems, you will continue to alter your bacteria in a negative way or damage the intestinal lining if you continue to feed them food that led to the altered flora or intestinal damage in the first place. A battle is waged between the probiotics and the altered gut flora from our diets. The winner is often disease and the probiotic manufacturers. We feel better while we're taking the probiotics, but symptoms promptly worsen when we discontinue them. No studies have been published that looked at correcting our diets with or without probiotics in a blinded fashion (one that controls for bias by having the investigator and the subject made unaware of whether one is consuming a placebo or the probiotic), so we don't really know whether just eating better foods would have derived the same benefits of the probiotics. These studies will probably never be performed (or at least published), since the companies that produce probiotics fund nearly all probiotic research, and there is no advantage to them to know whether dietary change is as beneficial as consuming their probiotic products.

What's worse is trying to sort out the probiotic data. While studies show potential benefit of certain bacterial strains of probiotics for one ailment, there is no "right" bacterial probiotic culture that treats all problems. Thus, this is where the confusion among physicians and the public arises. Let me give you an example. No less than three different probiotic bacteria (*Saccharomyces boulardii*, *Lactobacillus casei*, and *Lactobacillus rhamnosus*) have been shown to prevent antibiotic-associated diarrhea, while other strains of bacteria haven't shown any benefit. Additionally, some bacteria have been shown to help in the treatment of ulcerative colitis but not Crohn's disease. Both diseases are inflammatory conditions primarily involving the intestinal tract, yet some practitioners have recommended probiotics in the treatment of ulcerative colitis due to their established benefit but not so by others since they are costly and not covered by health insurance plans (Medicare or Medicaid). This is because the Food and Drug Administration considers them to be a dietary supplement, and as such, they don't regulate them. Dietary supplements aren't prescribed medications; hence, there is no coverage.

As I write this chapter, there are very specific examples, as I mentioned above, where probiotics are ready for prime time in treating ailments. The problem is that there is no regulatory control of their production. Until the Food and Drug Administration begins to regulate the science surrounding their use, it's difficult to convince many patients and physicians alike to consume an expensive "dietary supplement" for an indefinite amount of time, when many of the same bacteria are found in various yogurt preparations and can be consumed with a significantly lower financial impact. Additionally, many different strains of bacteria are generically labeled as probiotics, and most consumers and even health care providers are often confused as to which bacteria are beneficial for a specific ailment.

Probiotics are here to stay for conditions such as irritable bowel syndrome, infectious diarrhea, ulcerative colitis, and antibiotic use. We can quickly restore our intestinal flora after antibiotic use or recovery from an infection. We may add probiotics to our daily intake if we feel better while taking them, even if the science doesn't yet fully define their efficacy (irritable bowel syndrome, migraine headaches, type 2 diabetes, fatty liver, asthma, and so forth). Regardless, time will help us sort out what may be nothing more than a fad and what will truly be helpful for us. As we learn more about the gut flora and its interaction with disease and health, we will probably see more strains of probiotics with genuine medicinal qualities developed.

Pearls

- Probiotics may be beneficial in specific instances.
- Health plans don't cover them since they are considered a dietary supplement.

CHAPTER 20

The Lyons Lifestyle to Achieve Better Nutritional Health

Start by doing what's necessary; then do what's possible;
and suddenly you are doing the impossible.

Francis of Assisi

To get to this point in my understanding of our nutritional problems in America has been quite an undertaking. I'm beginning to understand the hole we've dug ourselves into by following flawed and outdated nutritional guidelines. These dietary guidelines have led us into worsening health across America. We now suffer from heart diseases, strokes, blood vessel diseases, cancers of all kinds, inflammatory diseases, autoimmune diseases, and dementia in epidemic proportions. We've seen an explosion of autism, suicide, depression, gallbladder disease, fatty liver disease, gastroesophageal reflux disease, high blood pressure, kidney failure, blood clots of the legs and lungs, and atrial fibrillation. Should we continue to follow the low-fat, high-carbohydrate, processed-food mantra of the last seventy years, or should we follow the science? Fortunately, we can make our own choices. In fact, we can make healthy nutritional decisions.

If you've read my other books or gotten this far in this book, you now realize that my only agenda is to teach you about the science concerning human metabolism as it relates to nutritional health. The guidance you and I were taught about nutrition and health is contradictory to what a mountain of medical science says. I first investigated the scientific literature about omega-3 and omega-6 fatty acid metabolism. This led to exploring trans fats and their devastating effects on metabolism and health. Once this very complex subject was clarified, I then tackled fructose. This, interestingly, was much easier to understand but a more difficult pill to swallow, since the Food and Drug Administration and the Department of Agriculture had convinced us to eat five servings of fruit per day. Fructose—"nature's candy bars," we were told—was quite natural, and so we bought into consuming fruit by the bucket load. To my chagrin, I now realize that eating five pieces of fruit is no different metabolically than eating five of my favorite candy bars each day. The metabolic effects are the same.

This book has continued on from where the first two books ended and moved my mind beyond thinking in a minimalistic fashion of just the effects of fats or fructose metabolism to looking at the big picture of a sound approach to improving our nutritional health. By continuing to study, take care of patients, and try to correct many of the health problems that affect them because of their bad nutrition, I have seen firsthand what has worked and where more has been required. The first big insight was when I systematically tried to reverse fatty liver disease.

Fatty liver disease is now the most common liver disease in America, and it didn't cause any significant problem in this country until the last quarter of the twentieth century. I first had patients stop consuming trans fats and placed them on omega-3 fatty acids. Many patients' livers normalized, but some continued to worsen. I then added my newfound understanding of fructose metabolism to those who continued to suffer from fatty liver, and again, many individuals improved with a reversal of metabolic syndrome by dramatically reducing this sugar from their diets. Finally, I now realize that exercise and reduced sugar intake from grains also play an important role in reducing fatty liver.

Not just one change is required to reverse fatty liver; it takes several steps and a commitment on our part to make those changes— not just for the moment but for a lifetime. My hope is that I have helped you understand why the changes are necessary without overwhelming you with too much science to boggle your mind. I also won't dumb it down so much that you won't see the importance of making those changes.

The following is a specific list of changes I believe are necessary to improve our health and possibly reverse some the damaging processes that may be in play. While I have continued to learn about many problems in our present nutritional guidelines, I will hopefully learn new insights in the future. I currently have seven Lyons Lifestyle recommendations that are straightforward and hopefully helpful to all of us.

1. Stop consuming all manufactured trans fats.
2. Increase your consumption of omega-3 fatty acids.
3. Decrease your intake of omega-6 fatty acids.
4. Dramatically decrease your fructose intake.
5. Decrease gluten and grain products.
6. Engage in a daily exercise routine several times per week.
7. Monitor your progress.

Let's look at these in detail.

1. **Stop consuming all manufactured trans fats.** These are the manufactured partially hydrogenated and hydrogenated fats found in processed foods. These modified vegetable oils are a major contributor to heart disease, stroke, and many cancers, which have exploded in the American population over the past

sixty years. As little as two hundred milligrams of trans fats per day are potentially toxic to the human body.

A. As I mentioned earlier in the book, the content of trans fat on the food label is a lie the Food and Drug Administration perpetuates. They authorized the food industry to label food products as zero grams of trans fat if the serving size contains less than five hundred milligrams. Labeling something as having zero grams trans fat per serving is not only misleading but also deceptive if consumers don't know about this manipulative labeling practice. All the producer needs to do is alter the serving size to fly under the radar rather than inform us of whether the product actually contains trans fats. Because of this little-known fact, you must look in the ingredient section of the food label. If that section reveals the presence of hydrogenated or partially hydrogenated vegetable oil, put the food product back on the shelf and find an alternative to consume or cook with.

B. Some of the more common grocery products that contain trans fats include Ritz crackers, Betty Crocker cake mixes, many tortillas, Coffee-Mate coffee creamer, some ice cream brands, many bakery items, and some condiments, to name a few. When in doubt, check the food label's ingredient section. Many alternatives now appear on the shelves of our supermarkets.

C. Hopefully, we may no longer see trans fats present at all, but that hasn't happened as of the publication of this book. The problem is that the food industry is in the process of developing a whole new group of fats (none found in nature) that will take the place of trans fats, and we don't yet know the medical consequences of any of these replacements. It would be best just to stick to nature's products rather than to switch to these new unknowns until we know the truth about them. These newly produced fats can be seen listed in the ingredient section of the food label and carry names such as fractionated palm oil, hydrogenated palm oil, and the like. We should avoid these fats until there is adequate data validating their safety.

2. **Increase your consumption of omega-3 fatty acids.** Our Western diet was pretty much stripped of this essential fatty acid by the end of the 1960s, but we've finally started to realize the devastating effects and are seeing the medical consequences of being deficient in this essential fat. While we know it's an essential nutrient for our health, there's still no guidance from the Food and Drug Administration, medical or nutritional organizations, or the World Health Organization about this requirement in our diets. They also haven't stressed the importance of its balance with omega-6 fatty acid consumption.

   A. Several cultures now consume very high quantities of omega-6 fats and suffer significant side effects. Because of that evidence, I believe we all need to find supplemental sources of this omega-3 fatty acid and consume it at least two times daily—at the start of our breakfast and during supper meals.

   B. Many foods contain omega-3 fatty acids. These include dark-green vegetables, fish and other seafood, grass- or greens-fed animal meat (cows, sheep, goats, and pigs), omega-3-enriched eggs from chickens fed flax or fish meal, unpasteurized milk from grass-fed cows or goats, wild game fowl and animals, flax meal, chia seeds, or quinoa seeds. Additionally, there is now an abundance of omega-3 fatty supplements found on the grocery store shelves. They provide an easy alternative to offer all of us an adequate alternative source of this essential fat.

C. It's always tough to know whether we're taking enough omega-3 fat in our diets. My goal is to consume at least two to three grams of omega-3 fat per day, and I divide this amount into at least two meals per day. The supplements on the store shelves that are the richest include flaxseed oil, fish oil, and krill oil.

D. You don't need a multi-omega (omega 3, 6, 9) supplement, since we consume excess omega-6 fatty acid and don't need omega-9 oil. The British government recommends thirty-five hundred milligrams of omega-3 fatty acids per day, while the United States suggests at least twenty-two hundred milligrams per day. But again, the Food and Drug Administration has established no recommended daily allowance at the time of this writing.

3. **Decrease your intake of omega-6 fatty acids.** Omega-6 fat consumption has dramatically increased in the last seventy-five years. This fat is the parent compound that induces inflammation and blood clotting. We now consume massive quantities of omega-6 fat from many sources in our diets.

A. Also known as linoleic acid, the primary sources are derived from seed and grain oils. The most prominent sources in our diets are corn oil, safflower oil, cottonseed oil, sunflower oil, peanut oil, processed soybean oil, and sesame oil.

B. Hydrogenated trans fats are primarily omega-6 fatty acids.

C. We clearly need to consume omega-6 fat to remain healthy, but the problem is that we need only about one to two grams per day, and we now consume up to forty-five grams of omega-6 fat daily in the Western diet. In the last half of the twentieth century, at the guidance of the federal government and nutritional and medical organizations, we moved away from the fats we had consumed for thousands of years. These included butterfat, tallow, lard, palm oil, coconut oil, and the like. These natural fats contain minimal amounts of omega-6 fat. My critical review of published data clearly shows that we should return to these fats, thereby dramatically reducing our omega-6 fat intake.

D. We shouldn't eliminate omega-6 fat from our diets, since it's essential to maintain nutritional health, but we need a balance between omega-3 and omega-6 fat intake, which has gone awry by present dietary guidelines.

E. No scientist today can acknowledge or defend the present guidance once he or she has studied all the data. It took several years of scientific inquiry to question the status quo, but the truth is slowly coming into view. Eating an egg isn't a problem if the chicken is fed flax or fish meal or is a free-range chicken; it is a problem if the chicken has been fed cornmeal. Grass-fed beef isn't a health problem; a cow fed corn silage is inflammatory to our bodies and creates an immunologic firestorm for us. We need to become aware of where we get our farm food. Unfortunately, the food industry produces farm food that is fed omega-6 foods (primarily corn and soy). We need to decrease our intake of foods fried in omega-6 oil. We need to decrease our intake of processed foods, since nearly all contain vegetable and seed oils rich in omega-6 oils.

F. Omega-3 fats cannot be used in any food product that has a long shelf life, since these oils oxidize and become rancid very quickly. Because of this fact, the processed food industry has used omega-6 fats since they have a long shelf life. Trans fats (partially hydrogenated or hydrogenated omega-6 vegetable oils) have an even longer shelf life. Saturated fats are very stable, but the problem with using them in processed foods is that the federal government has for so many decades told us they are dangerous for our health that it will take many years to reeducate the public about their safety. We were convinced to consume margarines, which uses omega-6 vegetable oils instead of butter. We were told not to eat other sources of saturated fats, as they would cause heart disease and strokes. Yet we now know that the mechanisms behind the cause of these diseases are from consuming excess amounts of omega-6 fat found in these vegetable and seed oils along with trans fats. The food label doesn't tell you how much omega-6 fat is contained in the foods you consume. Again, you must look in the ingredient section to see whether the microscopic list includes these oils. The bottom line is to decrease fried fast foods (all omega-6 or trans fats) and processed foods, and to stop cooking with most vegetable and seed oils.

G. If you're going to consume omega-6 oils as part of your meal (for example, fish-and-chips or corn-fed beefsteak), remember to take your omega-3 fat supplement before you start your meal to counter the effect of the omega-6 fat.

4. **Dramatically decrease fructose intake.** Nearly everyone loves sugar. We've also been convinced to consume large quantities of it surreptitiously. The hidden source of this sugar is fructose, which is found in fruit. Through hybridization and genetic modification in the last half century, we've seen a massive increase in sugar content of fruit. At the same time, the food pyramid and now the MyPlate advise us to eat massive quantities of fructose daily. This leads to an epidemic of metabolic syndrome (see chapter 5) in adults and the youth of America.

   A. The solution of guiding organizations and the federal government has been to focus on better diagnosis and treatment of the diseases of metabolic syndrome, eliminate soda pop from school vending machines, decrease salt intake, increase exercise, and the like. While none of these steps are necessarily bad, the problem is far bigger than this. I've seen thousands of patients reduce all sources of fructose, including fruit, fruit juice, honey, and sweets from sugar (50 percent fructose) and high-fructose corn syrup (45 to 55 percent fructose, depending on the food product). This change has dramatically improved problems with their health related to metabolic syndrome.

   B. Our livers contain a set of enzymes that need to be turned off to correct the metabolic syndrome occurring from daily, excess consumption of fructose. Studies show that it takes only six days to two weeks to turn on these enzymes (see my website at http://www.lyonsmedicalnews.com), and it also requires several weeks to turn them off. In fact, in some people who have been consuming excess sugar for several years, it may take up to a year for the normalization of hormones regulating their appetites after they've initiated a fructose fast. Fasting from fructose intake is a challenge for many of us, since the brain's effect from fructose leads to an "addicted" state, which requires about five to fourteen days of withdrawal before our cravings for sugar subside. Even after our hunger for sweets dissipates, we still have the task of turning off the liver enzymes that are driving fructose into the chemistry of the metabolic syndrome. That's why we need to continue to fast from fructose for several more days. Rarely the fast requires an extended amount of time if you're one of the unfortunate few who take up to a year for the normalization of the appetite hormones.

C. Fasting from all sources of fructose requires abstinence from all fruits and vegetables, and no consumption of juices, honey, pastries, pastas, breads, or cereals for three weeks. During that time you can consume any dairy products (except sweetened products like sweetened yogurt, chocolate milk, and so forth), meats (poultry, fish, and wild and domestic animals), and eggs.

D. Once the three weeks have passed, you can add back green vegetables since they are low in sugar. Sourdough bread contains no fructose and can be eaten after you've completed your fasting period. Be careful not to consume too much in the way of sugar beets, sweet corn, sweet potatoes, and sweet peas. They contain more fructose than other vegetables, and at this point, we don't want to open that enzyme pathway in the liver again if we can help it.

E. Fortunately, all we need to do is go through the fructose fast again to initiate closure of the liver enzyme pathway if we've overindulged in sugars for any length of time. Because we have so much fructose in our diets, I suggest that we go through a fast after the Christmas holidays and the summer fruit and berry season. We can easily indulge in excess fructose during these two times of the year, even if we do well with our diets during the rest of the year. As you add vegetables into your diet, you can also add a limited amount of starches and grains, but I will cover this more in the next point.

F. Suffice it to say, we need to learn to move away from the diet of the last fifty years and move back to a diet that will correct our metabolism and begin to reduce our risk of developing numerous diseases. Our typical consumption of fructose in 1960 was about ten grams per day. That is now around eighty-five grams per day. The food label doesn't contain any information about fructose content. My second book, *Fructose Exposed*, has twenty tables of foods showing how much fructose is present, and you need to learn how much fructose is present in the foods you regularly eat. Once you've learned this, modify your fructose accordingly. I haven't reproduced the tables in this book, but I would refer you to the ninth chapter of that book if you need help with this. Once you've lost your craving of sugar and your liver has shut down the metabolic syndrome enzyme pathway, pick a "treat" day every ten to fourteen days and eat whatever you choose. This breaks your psychological struggle with sweet deprivation and won't reactivate the liver enzyme pathway.

5. **Decrease gluten and grain products.** One of the most important additions to my first two books is the understanding I've gleaned from this problematic part of our diets. If we could return to the simple grains of the first half of the twentieth century, this wouldn't be an issue. But the sad fact is that through hybridization and genetic modification of our grains, we now have wheat consumption that is leading to celiac disease, diabetes, neurological disorders, obesity (see chapter 8), metabolic syndrome, and probably other disorders yet to be discovered. The breads, cakes, cookies, pizzas, pastas, and the like our grandmothers made for us aren't the food we're consuming today.

   A. Because of that, we either can go back to "old world" grains or need to dramatically decrease the intake of modern grains. Regardless, if we continue to consume the grain products we find in our bakeries and grocery stores, we will continue to suffer from their negative effects on our health. It's fascinating that both the food pyramid and now MyPlate guide our nutritional intake to consume several servings of grains per day in the form of cereals, breads, and the like. If we're to continue to follow their guidance, it would lead to many of the diseases we suffer from as a nation.

   B. Old-world grains are starting to be brought back to America. Farmers are beginning to realize that when we demand a better product to improve our nutritional health, they will have a market for their grains.

6. **Engage in a daily exercise routine several times per week.** My wife told me a while back that she wasn't convinced that there was any valid proof that exercise had any importance in the maintenance of our health. I embarked on investigating this area, since I have seen reports in the pediatric literature

that support her contentions when it comes to improved outcomes of managing diabetes, high blood pressure, and obesity in young people. What I did learn from my studies, though, is that an aerobic exercise program of twenty to thirty minutes per day for five to six days per week is beneficial for stimulating our metabolism to lose weight. Additionally, as we age, our muscle mass decreases, and exercise that increases muscle strength a couple of times per week sustains and/or increases that muscle mass.

A. Exercise is helpful in reducing falls, hip fractures, and the like. The older we get, the more important this clearly becomes, as studies have repeatedly demonstrated. Running a marathon or triathlon isn't necessary, but even activities such as bowling, working in the garden, going for a brisk walk, performing household chores, or raking leaves in the yard (the list is endless) are all very beneficial and don't require an expensive membership to a local gym. Aerobic exercise and muscle strengthening can be combined as well, and we derive benefit from both activities simultaneously with activities such as doing yoga, dancing, swimming, playing a round of golf, gardening, and the like. An integral part of exercise is to maintain our weight in a reasonable range.

B. Modern data show that total body weight isn't as important as belly fat. Men need to reduce their waistlines to be smaller than forty inches, and women less than thirty-five inches. If you aren't sure of your waist size, just measure it. As we've learned, the bulge is directly related to excess carbohydrate intake. The biggest culprits are fructose-containing products; the big five are fruit, fruit juice, honey, products sweetened with table sugar, and products that contain high-fructose corn syrup. The other big sources of carbohydrates are grains (cereals, breads, pastas, pastries, pizzas, and so forth) and starches (rice, potatoes, and so forth). If we ate only potatoes or rice at supper, it wouldn't be a big deal. Likewise, a bowl of oat cereal for breakfast isn't a problem. But we now consume several servings of fructose-containing foods as well as grains and starches several times every day, and we cannot adequately metabolize all these carbohydrates.

C. We don't have the metabolism of herbivores, but the guidance of federal government agencies and medical and nutritional organizations strongly encourages us to eat this way. The metabolic consequences have been devastating, to say the least. Obesity, the diseases caused by metabolic syndrome, cancer, and inflammatory and autoimmune diseases now plague most of us because of our diets. Reducing our weight to a moderate range and eliminating belly fat are critical to improving our health. This is done by both exercising and reducing carbohydrate intake. The more vigorous we exercise, the more carbohydrates we can ingest and get away with. But as we age, our metabolic rate slows, our activity level diminishes, and our caloric demands fall. Unfortunately, we often continue to consume too many calories, and so we begin to gain weight. Most calories are derived from the various carbohydrates we mentioned. Combining exercise with carbohydrate reduction will lead to weight loss and improved metabolism.

7. **Monitor your progress.** When I was a young doctor, we knew very little about the causes of viral hepatitis. In the past

thirty-five years, many viruses have been identified, and our knowledge about infectious hepatitis now fills entire textbooks. Likewise, when we first began monitoring the health of our bodies, we could perform a physical examination, measure blood pressure, perform some blood tests, and on occasion obtain tests such as a chest x-ray or electrocardiogram. As we are learning about the markers for disease risk, presence, or progression, we're now developing tests that can monitor our metabolic state, cancer risk, and the like. We now have blood tests that measure our lipid profile, liver enzymes, and degree of inflammation present in our bodies. Soon we will be able to measure the omega-3 and omega-6 content in our bodies (this is already being done in research and is commercially available, but our insurance plans do not yet cover it). We're developing the laboratory tools to monitor our bodies' progress in reversing the damage that has occurred because of our diets. Regardless, it's currently easy to have your health care provider check your lipid profile, inflammation markers, fasting insulin, and glycosylated hemoglobin levels (for possible diabetes) and liver enzymes (for fatty liver). Measuring your waistline is also easy.

A. Laboratory tests should be done initially before and then three to six months after implementing your lifestyle changes. The blood tests will track your progress.

B. Additionally, available blood tests can screen you for the risk of celiac disease, but they need to be obtained before you eliminate gluten from your diet, as the blood test may be negative if you've been avoiding it for a few months before you get tested. If your antibodies for celiac disease are positive, a gastroenterologist should evaluate you.

C. Finally, and most importantly, if you're taking medications to treat the maladies related to your diet, you need to seek help from your physician to monitor your blood sugar, blood pressure, liver function, lipid panel, and the like, since you may need to reduce or eliminate some of your medications as your metabolic profile improves and you lose weight.

Pearls

- Adopting the seven-point Lyons Lifestyle will improve your nutritional health.
- The Lyons Lifestyle is a way of life, not a fad diet plan.

CHAPTER 21

Concluding Thoughts

The least initial deviation from the truth is
multiplied later a thousand fold.

Aristotle

If you've ever been driving at night in a snowstorm and turned your
headlights on high beam, suddenly your vision dramatically worsens.
The glare of light bouncing off the snowflakes can reduce your visibility
to just a few feet in front of your car. If you quickly revert back to low
beam, your sight promptly improves.

After I completed writing my first book, which reveals the
devastating effects of trans fats and the importance of balancing our
omega-3 and omega-6 fat intake, I felt like I was driving through the
storm on low beams. Prior to studying fat physiology to the depth of
my present understanding, I had been driving in the dark without even
having my headlights on. The decade of intense study that culminated
in *42 Days to a New Life* had turned on my headlights, since I came
to understand how our diets had changed for the worse during the
first half of the twentieth century. For a short period of time, I felt as
though I was beginning to understand why many of us have acquired
the chronic medical problems that plague America because of trans fats

and an imbalance of the essential fats (omega-3 and omega-6) that had evolved in the Western diet.

I was immediately forced back onto the high beam, and my vision worsened when I was challenged to find out why high-fructose corn syrup was "killing" us. That led to my second book, *Fructose Exposed*, which explored the consequences of daily consuming excess fructose. The pattern of high fructose intake is now standard for the uneducated, and we can see its disastrous effects on millions every day. We started getting fat and developing the metabolic syndrome as we increased our fructose intake by nearly 800 percent over the past half century.

I developed guidelines for my patients and instantly saw benefits in those who complied. The recommendations were simple and straightforward but difficult to accomplish for some individuals. The activated metabolism that occurs related to excess, daily fructose ingestion causes addiction to carbohydrates that can be quite challenging to withdraw from. Once fructose ingestion has been discontinued for a couple of weeks, our bodies slowly begin to reverse the created metabolic mess. As patients get control of their carbohydrate intake and no longer crave sugar, they can see the benefits of weight loss, increased energy, and a decrease in medication needs. Their laboratory values improve, and they slowly see the reappearance of their waistlines. I was feeling pretty good at this juncture. I thought that, between the two books, I had accomplished much to help my patients.

Back on low beam, with better "vision" again, I thought I was finally getting a handle on the medical problems our diets had caused. Pow! The blinding light came right back when I continued my studies. I continued to gain better insight and confirmation of the conclusions of my first two books, but new information exposed other major issues brewing in our diets that needed to be brought to light. Hence, this research led to the writing of this book. The diagrams and data found in the first books haven't significantly changed since their respective publications, so refer to them for specifics on the fructose and fat content of foods.

In this book I tried to develop some basic guidelines to follow that will serve you nutritionally to prevent or reverse medical problems that have been a direct result of your diet. Additionally, I have updated the concepts outlined in those editions.

Prior to 1993, when I started my first project on fats in our diets, I was clearly driving in the dark. I didn't even have my headlights on and had no idea where I was going. I was busy in my gastroenterology practice while attending meetings and learning the latest treatments, tests, and procedures in an attempt to take care of my patients. I didn't stop and question why we were all getting sicker. Rather, I was just trying to provide my patients with the most up-to-date care modern medicine provides.

Whether I would have begun to investigate any of these subjects and write about them on my own, I will never know. But I am truly thankful for the nurse who suggested that I find out why flaxseed oil changed her life and solved her medical problems in 1993. Once the headlights came on, my research has been on a high beam/low beam ritual in the snowstorm. At first, I couldn't see anything, but then things started to sort themselves out. Then I realized I knew only part of the story, and I was back on the high beams. The completion of this book makes me want to conclude that I'm on low beams. The question is, for how long?

You and I know that our world of knowledge is growing at an exponential pace. I'm sure it won't be long before the high beams come back on. My patients seem to find a way to prompt that effect in me.

My goal in writing this book was to provide you with the most recent nutritional insights behind the problems created by the Western diet. As we consume fats and sugars from various food sources, as the Food and Drug Administration, the Department of Agriculture, the Department of Health and Human Services, the American Heart

Association, the American Dietetic Association, and the World Health Organization (to name some specifically) suggest, knowing what is detrimental and beneficial to our nutritional health is confusing. We've been told to consume three to five servings of fruit per day, yet that diet will lead to metabolic syndrome in most of us. We are told to eat an abundance of grains, but this practice has led to obesity, celiac/gluten problems, and so forth. We are told to avoid saturated fats and consume grain and seed oils, but this routine has inflamed our bodies and led to a multitude of medical problems. We've included manufactured trans fats in our diets, reduced our intake of saturated fats and cholesterol, and turned to vegetable oils rich in omega-6 fat.

But now millions of us are plagued by vitamin D deficiency, gastroesophageal reflux disease, fatty liver disease, kidney disease, autoimmune diseases, mental disorders, cancers, and heart disease. We have no official guidance on omega-3 fat consumption, and a recommended daily allowance for this essential fat hasn't been defined. What's worse, pasteurization and homogenization of milk and the removal of cod liver oil from our diets have led to omega-3 fat deficiency in America. We changed farm animal food from grass to corn and soy-based foods, and animals have lost their omega-3 fat and consumed excess omega-6 fat. This shift has led to sick farm animals and an ever-increasing need for antibiotics and hormones to get them to the butcher before they die.

I'll never convince myself that any of the changes leading to drastic transformations in our diets were part of a "conspiracy" to make us sick. My belief is that most changes at the time they occurred were altruistic. Attempts were made to increase the shelf life of food with the addition of trans fat to these products so fewer people would go hungry. Hybridization and genetic modification led to a significant increase in the yield in food production. Again, this measure would provide more food for the planet.

Pasteurization of milk was reportedly mandated to decrease the incidence of tuberculosis, which can be transferred to humans when consuming unpasteurized milk. The sad story here is that we had been drinking raw milk for millennia, and tuberculosis was on a rapid decline after World War I once modern dairy hygiene practices were implemented. Pasteurization wasn't implemented nationally until 1962, and the problem with tuberculosis was nearly nonexistent by that time. The consequences of mandated pasteurization were unforeseen, but we are only now realizing just how poor that decision turned out to be.

There is more vitamin C in a glass of unpasteurized milk than in an orange. Pasteurization destroys not only omega-3 fatty acids but also all water-soluble vitamins, including vitamin C. This again led to intervention with massive expansion of the fruit industry, the development of the food pyramid and now MyPlate promoting fruit consumption. I don't think there was an intention in this country to create obesity or metabolic syndrome in seventy million adults and millions of our youth; rather, we were trying to promote economics and "natural" agribusiness.

Finally, we developed a policy for corn production in the 1970s that allowed us to produce sugar cheaply in the form of high-fructose corn syrup. We're now paying the medical price for that decision, with the rapid rise of metabolic syndrome and its consequences now afflicting nearly one-third of the US population. While we made interventions and changes to our food supply for "noble" purposes, it's very clear to me at this point that the consequences of those changes led to harmful outcomes in our health as a nation.

Health care now consumes one-sixth of our economy. Isn't it ironic that when I was a child, my parents didn't have health insurance? None of us needed health insurance. None of us were suffering from heart disease or dying from cancer. And the cost of health care was low enough that it was a cash-and-carry proposition for Mom and Dad. I was hospitalized in the third grade for pneumonia, but it didn't bankrupt my parents. They just paid for it. My brother needed his tonsils removed. The procedure didn't break the bank. Another brother broke his collarbone and needed medical care. We got by without health insurance.

Today that situation would be out of the question because we're now all destined to so many chronic diseases that require constant monitoring, daily medications, and expensive testing and interventions for their complications. None of the maladies that affected my brothers or me were a chronic problem. It's the chronic diseases caused by our diets that have driven up the cost of health care to the tune of $500 billion annually just for big medication costs to address those chronic ailments.

For us to have an impact on the exorbitant health care costs consuming American dollars and dividing this country politically, we need to get control of what we consume in our daily diets. By following the guidelines I've outlined in this book, you can begin to improve your health, reduce the need for excessive medical testing, decrease or eliminate the need for chronic medications, and possibly reduce your need for very expensive treatments, such as cancer therapy, heart stenting, gallbladder removal, hiatal hernia repair to stop acid reflux, and the like.

Knowledge truly empowers us to have better control of our lives. This book tries to give you that power. Misinformation perpetuated ever since the six-country study in the early 1950s led to exploitation of America in a way that will never be truly known. Additionally, our failure to react to the scientific proof that trans fat ingestion is the primary cause of heart disease and cancer in the late 1950s has led to untold numbers of individuals who suffered and/or died prematurely. Mandated pasteurization and homogenization of milk destroyed its intrinsic goodness. Adopting the low-fat, high-carbohydrate diet as our American diet has led to failing nutritional health. It's the worst diet on the planet, as numerous prospective studies now document. It's finally time to abandon these antiquated dietary guidelines and revert to the diet of my grandmother. This is the foundation of the Lyons Lifestyle for better nutritional health.

Driving in a blinding snowstorm or knowing what to carry home from the grocery store can all be rather burdensome. I hope this book has laid the foundation for you so you can see things a bit more clearly concerning the latter. I'm sure this much information packed into one book might seem a bit overwhelming, but I believe with motivated effort on your part, it will greatly assist you in making better choices about your nutrition-related health. Consider the Lyons Lifestyle choice. Best of luck!

I've included this table to show you what the various fats and sugars I've discussed in this book do to our blood chemistry as well as their associated risks with heart disease (CAD) and cancer. I hope this is a helpful synopsis for you. At the bottom of the table is the ideal effect that would reduce our heart disease and cancer risk.

	HDL	Neutral LDL	"Bad" LDL	Triglycerides	CRP	Uric Acid	Insulin Resist	CAD Risk	Cancer Risk
Trans Fats	Reduces		Increases	Increases	Increases		Increases	Increases	Increases
Omega-3 Fats	Increases		Reduces	Reduces				Reduces	Reduces
Omega-6 Fats	Reduces			Increases	Increases			Increases	Increases
Saturated Fats	Increases	Raises	Reduces	Reduces			Reduces	Reduces	Reduces
Daily Excess Fructose	Reduces		Increases	Increases		Increases	Increases	Increases	
Daily Excess Glucose							Increases	Increases	
Olive Oil (Omega-9)	No Change	Doesn't Matter	Reduces						
Low fat, Vegan Diet	Reduces		Reduces	Increases					
Low Sat'd Fat Diet							Increases	Increases	Increases
IDEAL EFFECT	INCREASES	DOESN'T MATTER	REDUCES	REDUCES	REDUCES	REDUCES	REDUCES	REDUCES	REDUCES

BIBLIOGRAPHY

Abd El-Kader, S. M., and E. M. Salah El-Den Ashmawy. "Nonalcoholic Fatty Liver Disease: The Diagnosis and Management." *World Journal of Hepatology* 7 (2015): 846–58.

Amara, A. A., and A. Shibl. "Role of Probiotics in Health Improvement, Infection Control, and Disease Treatment and Management." *Saudi Pharmaceutical Journal* 23 (2015): 107–14.

An, W. S., S. M. Lee, Y. K. Son, et al. "Omega-3 Fatty Acid Supplementation Increases 1,25-Dihydroxyvitamin D and Fetuin-A Levels in Dialysis Patients." *Nutrition Research* 32 (2012): 495–502.

Anderson, A. K., D. M. McDougald, and M. Steiner-Asiedu. "Dietary Trans-Fatty Acid Intake and Maternal and Infant Adiposity." *European Journal of Clinical Nutrition* 64 (2010): 1308–15.

Anderson, J. T., F. Grande, and A. Keys. "Hydrogenated Fats in the Diet and Lipids in the Serum of Man." *Journal of Nutrition* 75 (1961): 368–94.

Andrews J. S., W. H. Griffith, J. F. Mead, and R. A. Stein. "Toxicity of Air-Oxidized Soybean Oil." *Journal of Nutrition* 70 (1960): 199–210.

Appel, L. J., F. M. Sacks, V. J. Carey, et al. "OmniHeart Collaborative Research Group. Effects of Protein, Monounsaturated Fat, and Carbohydrate Intake on Blood Pressure and Serum Lipids: Results of the OmniHeart Randomized Trial." *Journal of the American Medical Association* 294 (2003): 2455–64.

Appleton, K. M., P. J. Rogers, and A. R. Ness. "Updated Systematic Review and Meta-analysis of the Effects of N-3 Long-Chain Polyunsaturated Fatty Acids on Depressed Mood." *American Journal of Clinical Nutrition* 91 (2010): 75–770.

Aravanis, C. "The Classic Risk Factors for Coronary Heart Disease: Experience in Europe." *Preventive Medicine* 12 (1983): 16–19.

Aro, A., M. Jauhiainen, R. Partanen, I. Saminen, and M. Mutanen. "Steric Acid, Trans-Fatty Acids, and Dairy Fat: Effects on Serum and Lipoprotein Lipids, Apolipoproteins, Lipoprotein A, and Lipid Transfer Proteins in Healthy Subjects." *American Journal of Clinical Nutrition* 65 (1997): 1419–26.

Aro, A., I. Salminen, J. K. Huttunen, et al. "Adipose Tissue Isomeric Trans-Fatty Acids and Risk of Myocardial Infarction in Nine Countries: The EURAMIC Study." *Lancet* 345 (1995): 273–78.

Ascherio, A., M. B. Katan, P. L. Zock, et al. "Trans-Fatty Acids and Coronary Heart Disease." *New England Journal of Medicine* 340 (1999): 1994–98.

Astorg, P. "Dietary Fatty Acids and Colorectal and Prostate Cancers: Epidemiological Studies." *Bulletin of Cancer* 92 (2005): 670–84.

Astrup, A., J. Dyerberg, P. Elwood, et al. "The Role of Reducing Intakes of Saturated Fat in the Prevention of Cardiovascular Disease: Where Does the Evidence Stand in 2010?" *American Journal of Clinical Nutrition* 93 (2010): 684–88.

Austin, G. L., M. T. Thiny, E. C. Westman, W. S. Yancy, and N. J. Shaheen. "A Very Low-Carbohydrate Diet Improves Gastroesophageal Reflux and Its Symptoms." *Digestive Disease and Sciences* 51 (2006): 1307–12.

Autier, P., M. Boniol, C. Pizot, and P. Mullie. "Vitamin D Status and Ill Health: A Systematic Review." *Lancet Diabetes and Endocrinology* 2 (2013): 76–89.

Beaglehole, R., M. A. Foulkes, I. A. M. Prior, and E. F. Eyles. "Cholesterol and Mortality in New Zealand Maoris." *British Medical Journal* 280 (1980): 285–87.

Biesalski, H. K. "Meat and Cancer: Meat as a Component of a Healthy Diet." *European Journal of Nutrition and Metabolism* 56 (2002): S2–S11.

Blackburn, G. L. "Mechanisms of Nitrogen Sparing with Severe Calorie Restricted Diets." *International Journal of Obesity* 5 (1981): 215–16.

Boden, G., K. Sargrad, C. Homko, et al. "Effect of a Low-Carbohydrate Diet on Appetite, Blood Glucose Levels, and Insulin Resistance in Obese Patients with Type 2 Diabetes." *Annals of Internal Medicine* 142 (2005): 403–11.

Broad, W. J. "NIH Deals Gingerly with Diet-Disease Link." *Science* 204 (1979): 1175–78.

Brymora, A., M. Flisinski, R. J. Johnson, et al. "Low-Fructose Diet Lowers Blood Pressure and Inflammation in Patients with Chronic Kidney Disease." *Nephrology, Dialysis, and Transplantation* 27 (2012): 608–12.

Byers, T. "Hardened Fats, Hardened Arteries?" *New England Journal of Medicine* 337 (1997): 1544–45.

Caballero, B., T. Clay, S. M. Davis, et al. "Pathways: A School-Based, Randomized Controlled Trial for the Prevention of Obesity in American Indian Schoolchildren." *American Journal of Clinical Nutrition* 78 (2003): 1030–38.

Calder, P. C. "Polyunsaturated Fatty Acids and Inflammation." *Biochemical Society Transactions* 33 (2005): 423–27.

Campos, H., et al. "LDL Particle Size Distribution: Results from the Framingham Offspring Study." *Arteriosclerosis and Thrombosis* 12 (1992): 1410–19.

Cao, L., L. Wang, L. Yang, et al. "Long-Term Effect of Early-Life Supplementation with Probiotics on Preventing Atopic Dermatitis: A Meta-Analysis." *Journal of Dermatological Treatment* (May 5, 2015): 1–4.

Caselli, M., F. Cassol, G. Calo, et al. "Actual Concept of 'Probiotics': Is It More Functional to Science or Business?" *World Journal of Gastroenterology* 19 (2013): 1527–40.

Cassady, B. A., N. L. Charboneau, E. E. Brys, K. A. Crouse, D. C. Beitz, and T. Wilson. "Effects of Low-Carbohydrate Diets in Red Meats or Poultry, Fish, and Shellfish on Plasma Lipids and Weight Loss." *Nutrition and Metabolism* 4 (2007): 23, doi:10.1186/1743-7075-4-23.

Cassidy, A., V. I. De Vivo, Y. Liu, et al. "Associations between Diet, Lifestyle Factors, and Telomere Length in Women." *American Journal of Clinical Nutrition* 91 (2010): 1273–80.

Castelli, W. P. "Concerning the Possibility of a Nut." *Journal of the American Medical Association* 152 (1992): 1371–72.

Chajes, V., A. C. M. Thiebaut, M. Rotival, et al. "Association between Serum Trans-Monounsaturated Fatty Acids and Breast Cancer Risk in the E3N-EPIC Study." *American Journal of Epidemiology* 167 (2008): 1312–20.

Charbonneau, B., H. M. O'Connor, A. H. Wang, et al. "Trans-Fatty Acid Intake Is Associated with Increased Risk and N-3 Fatty Acid Intake with Reduced Risk of Non-Hodgkin Lymphoma." *Journal of Nutrition* 143 (2013): 672–81.

Chavarro J. E., M. J. Stampfer, H. Campos, et al. "A Prospective Study of Trans-Fatty Acid Levels in Blood and Risk of Prostate Cancer." *Cancer Epidemiology, Biomarkers, and Prevention* 17 (2008): 95–101.

Cheung, O., A. Kapoor, P. Puri, et al. "The Impact of Fat Distribution on the Severity of Nonalcoholic Fatty Liver Disease and Metabolic Syndrome." *Hepatology* 46 (2007): 1091–100.

Chowdhury, R., S. Warnakula, S. Kunutsor, et al. "Association of Dietary, Circulating, and Supplement Fatty Acids with Coronary Risk." *Annals of Internal Medicine* 160 (2014): 398–406.

Church, T. S., J. L. Kuk, R. Ross, et al. "Association of Cardiorespiratory Fitness, Body Mass Index, and Waist Circumference to Nonalcoholic Fatty Liver Disease." *Gastroenterology* 130 (2006): 2023–30.

Ciorba, M. A. "A Gastroenterologist's Guide to Probiotics." *Clinical Gastroenterology and Hepatology* 10 (2010): 960–68.

Conklin S. M., J. I. Harris, S. B. Manuck, et al. "Serum Omega-3 Fatty Acids Are Associated with Variation in Mood, Personality, and Behavior in Hypercholesterolemic Community Volunteers." *Psychiatry Research* 152 (2007): 1–10.

Cox, C. L., K. L. Stanhope, J. M. Schwartz, et al. "Consumption of Fructose but Not Glucose-Sweetened Beverages for 10 Weeks Increases Circulating Concentrations of Uric Acid, Retinol Binding Protein-4, and Gamma-Glutamyl Transferase Activity in Overweight/Obese Humans." *Nutrition and Metabolism* 9 (2012): 68.

Crampton, E. W., R. H. Common, E. T. Pritchard, and F. A. Farmer. "Studies to Determine the Nature of the Damage to the Nutritive Value of Some Begetable Oils from Heat Treatment: IV. Ethyl Esters of Heat Polymerized Linseed, Soybean, and Sunflower Seed Oils." *Journal of Nutrition* 60 (1956): 13–24.

Culling K. S., H. A. Neil, M. Gilbert, and K. N. Frayn. "Effects of Short-Term Low- and High-Carbohydrate Diets on Postprandial Metabolism in Nondiabetic and Diabetic Subjects." *Nutrition, Metabolism, and Cardiovascular Disease* 19 (2009): 345–51.

Dawber, T. R., R. J. Nickerson, F. N. Brand, and J. Pool. "Eggs, Serum Cholesterol, and Coronary Heart Disease." *American Journal of Clinical Nutrition* 36 (1982): 617–25.

Dawson-Hughes, B., S. S. Harris, A. H. Lichtenstein, et al. "Dietary Fat Increase Vitamin D-3 Absorption." *Journal of the Academy of Nutrition and Dietetics* 115 (2015): 225–30.

Dawson-Hughes, B., S. S. Harris, N. J. Palermo, et al. "Meal Conditions Affect the Absorption of Supplemental Vitamin D3 but Not the Plasma 25-Hydroxyvitamin D Response to Supplementation." *Journal of Bone and Mineral Research* 28 (2013): 1778–83.

Didari, T., S. Mozaffari, S. Nikfar, and M. Abdollahi. "Effectiveness of Probiotics in Irritable Bowel Syndrome: Updated Systematic Review with Meta-Analysis." *World Journal of Gastroenterology* 21 (2015): 3072–84.

Dietary Guidelines Advisory Committee. "Scientific Report of the 2015 Dietary Guidelines Advisory Committee." Accessed January 20, 2016. http://www.health.gov/dietaryguidelines/2015-scientific-report/.

Dreon, D. M., H. A. Fernstrom, P. T. Williams, and R. M. Krauss. "A Very Low-Fat Diet Is Not Associated with Improved Lipoprotein Profiles in Men with a Predominance of Large, Low-Density Lipoproteins." *American Journal of Clinical Nutrition* 69 (1999): 411–18.

Dyerberg, S. J., and A. N. Astrup. "High Levels of Industrially Produced Trans Fat in Popular Fast Foods." *New England Journal of Medicine* 354 (2006): 1650–52.

Eckel, R. H., J. M. Jakicic, V. S. Hubbard, et al. "Guideline on Lifestyle Management to Reduce Cardiovascular Risk: A Report of the American College of Cardiology/American Heart Association Task Force on Practice Guidelines." *Circulation* 2013, doi:10.1161/01. cir.0000437740.48606.d1.

Egert, S., F. Kannenberg, V. Somoza, et al. "Dietary Alpha-Linolenic Acid, EPA, and DHA Have Differential Effects on LDL Fatty

Acid Composition but Similar Effects on Serum Lipid Profiles in Normolipidemic Humans." *Journal of Nutrition* 139 (2009): 861–68.

Eliades, M., and E. Spyrou. "Vitamin D: A New Player in Nonalcoholic Fatty Liver Disease?" *World Journal of Gastroenterology* 21 (2015): 1718–27.

Elias, P. K., et al. "Serum Cholesterol and Cognitive Performance in the Framingham Heart Study." *Psychosomatic Medicine* 67 (2005): 24–30.

Emond, M. J., and W. Zareba. "Prognostic Value of Cholesterol in Women of Different Ages." *Journal of Women's Health* 6 (197): 295–307.

Enig, M. G. *Know Your Fats: The Complete Primer for Understanding the Nutrition of Fat, Oils, and Cholesterol.* Silver Spring, MD: Bethesda, 2000.

Enig, M. G. *Trans-Fatty Acids in the Food Supply: A Comprehensive Report Covering 60 Years of Research.* 2nd ed. Silver Spring, MD: Enig Associates, 1995.

Enig M. G., S. Atal, M. Keeney, and J. Sampugna. "Isomeric Trans-Fatty Acids in the US Diet." *Journal of American College of Nutrition* 9 (1990): 471–86.

Enig, M. G., R. Munn, and M. Keeney. "Dietary Fat and Cancer Trends: A Critique." *Federation Proceedings* 37 (1978): 2215–220.

Esterbauer, H., R. J. Schaur, and H. Zollner. "Autoxidation of Human Low Density Lipoprotein: Loss of Polyunsaturated Fatty Acids and Vitamin E and Generation of Aldehydes." *Free Radical Biology and Medicine* 11 (1991): 81–128.

Estruch, R., E. Ros, J. Salas-Salvado, et al. "PREDIMED Study Investigators. Primary Prevention of Cardiovascular Disease with a Mediterranean Diet." *New England Journal of Medicine* 368 (2013): 1279–90.

Farzaneh-Far, R., W. S. Harris, S. Garg, et al. "Inverse Association of Erythrocyte N-3 Fatty Acid Levels with Inflammatory Biomarkers in Patients with Stable Coronary Artery Disease: The Heart and Soul Study." *Atherosclerosis* 205 (2009): 538–43.

Feinleib, M. "On a Possible Inverse Relationship between Serum Cholesterol and Cancer Mortality." *American Journal of Epidemiology* 114 (1982): 5–10.

Feinleib, M. "Summary of a Workshop on Cholesterol and Noncardiovascular Disease Mortality." *Preventive Medicine* 11 (1982): 360–67.

Ferlay, A., M. Doreau, C. Martin, and Y. Chilliard. "Effects of Incremental Amounts of Extruded Linseed on the Milk Fatty Acid Composition of Dairy Cows Receiving Hay or Corn Silage." *Journal of Dairy Science* 96 (2013): 6577–595.

Ferro-Luzzi, A., and F. Branca. "Mediterranean Diet, Italian-Style: Prototype of a Healthy Diet." *American Journal of Clinical Nutrition* 61 (1995): 1338S–1345S.

Fontani, G., F. Corradeschi, A. Felici, et al. "Cognitive and Physiological Effects of Omega-3 Polyunsaturated Fatty Acid Supplementation in Healthy Subjects." *European Journal of Clinical Investigation* 35 (2005): 691–99.

Forsythe, C. E., S. D. Phinney, R. D. Feinman, et al. "Limited Effect of Dietary Saturated Fat on Plasma Saturated Fat in the Context of a Low-Carbohydrate Diet." *Lipids* 45 (2010): 947–157.

Foster, G. D., H. R. Wyatt, J. O. Hill, et al. "Weight and Metabolic Outcomes after 2 Years on a Low-Carbohydrate Diet: A Randomized Trial." *Annals of Internal Medicine* 153 (2010): 147–57.

Ferrucci, L., A. Cherubini, S. Bandinelli, et al. "Relationship of Plasma Polyunsaturated Fatty Acids to Circulating Inflammatory Markers." *Journal of Clinical Endocrinology and Metabolism* 91 (2006): 439–46.

Fox, M., C. Barr, S. Nolan, et al. "The Effects of Dietary Fat and Calorie Density on Esophageal Acid Exposure and Reflux Symptoms." *Clinical Gastroenterology and Hepatology* 5 (2007): 439–44.

Garcia-Palmieri, M. R., P. D. Sorlie, R. Costas, and R. J. Havlik. "An Apparent Inverse Relationship between Serum Cholesterol and Cancer Mortality in Puerto Rico." *American Journal of Epidemiology* 114 (1981): 29–40.

Gardner C. D., A. Kiazand, S. Alhassan, et al. "Comparison of the Atkins, Zone, Ornish and LEARN Diets for Change in Weight and Related Risk Factors among Overweight Premenopausal Women: The A-to-Z Weight-Loss Study: A Randomized Trial." *Journal of the American Medical Association* 297 (2007): 969–77.

Geliebter, A., C. N. Ochner, C. L. Dambkowski, and S. A. Hashim. "Obesity-Related Hormones and Metabolic Risk Factors: A Randomized Trial of Diet plus Either Strength or Aerobic Training versus Diet Alone in Overweight Participants." *Journal of Diabetes and Obesity* 29 (2014): 1–7.

German, J. B., R. A. Gibson, R. M. Krauss, et al. "A Reappraisal of the Impact of Dairy Foods and Milk Fat on Cardiovascular Disease Risk." *European Journal of Nutrition* 48 (2009): 191–203.

Ghouri, Y. A., D. M. Richards, E. F. Rahimi, et al. "Systematic Review of Randomized Controlled Trials of Probiotics, Prebiotics, and Synbiotics in Inflammatory Bowel Disease." *Clinical and Experimental Gastroenterology* 7 (2014): 473–87.

GianMarco G., G. Brandimarte, F. Fabiocchi, et al. "Interactions between Innate Immunity, Microbiota, and Probiotics." *Journal of Immunology Research* 2015, doi:10.1155/2015/501361.

Gillman, M. W., et al. "Inverse Association of Dietary Fat with the Development of Ischemic Stroke in Men." *Journal of the American Medical Association* 278 (1997): 2145–150.

Glueck, C. J. "Appraisal of Dietary Fat as a Causative Factor in Atherogenesis." *American Journal of Clinical Nutrition* 32 (1979): 2637–2631.

Golomb, B. A., M. E. Evans, H. L. White, and J. E. Dimsdale. "Trans Fat Consumption and Aggression." *PLoS One* 7:e32175, 2012.

Gordon, R. S., and A. Cherrkes. "Unesterified Fatty Acid in Human Blood Plasma." *Journal of Clinical Investigation* 35 (1956): 206–12

Greenberg, S. M., and A. C. Frazer. "Some Factors Affecting the Growth and Development of Rats Fed Rancid Fat." *Journal of Nutrition* 50 (1953): 421–40.

Greenblatt, J. M. "Low Cholesterol and Its Psychological Effects: Low Cholesterol Is Linked to Depression, Suicide, and Violence." *Psychology Today*, June 10, 2011.

Guberan, E. "Surprising Decline of Cardiovascular Mortality in Switzerland: 1951–1976." *Journal of Epidemiology and Community Health* 33 (1979): 114–20.

Hansen, C. P., T. L. Berentzen, J. Halkjaer, et al. "Intake of Ruminant Trans-Fatty Acids and Changes in Body Weight and Waist Circumference." *European Journal of Clinical Nutrition* 66 (2012): 1104–09.

Harper, A. "Dietary Goals: A Skeptical View." *American Journal of Clinical Nutrition* 31 (1978): 310–21.

Harvey, K. A., C. L. Walker, Z Xu, et al. "Trans-Fatty Acids: Induction of a Pro-inflammatory Phenotype in Endothelial Cells." *Lipids* 47 (2012): 647–57.

Hays, J. H., A. DiSabitino, R. T. Gorman, S. Vincent, and M. E. Stillabower. "Effect of a High-Saturated Fat and No-Starch Diet on Serum Lipid Subfractions in Patients with Documented Atherosclerotic Cardiovascular Disease." *Mayo Clinic Proceedings* 78 (2003): 1331–36.

Hession M., C. Rolland, U. Kulkarni, A. Wise, and J. Broom. "Systematic Review of Randomized Controlled Trials of Low-Carbohydrate vs. Low-Fat/Low-Calorie Diets in the Management of Obesity and Its Comorbidities." *Obesity Reviews* 10 (2009): 36–50.

Hibbeln, J. R., and N. Salem Jr. "Dietary Polyunsaturated Fatty Acids and Depression: When Cholesterol Does Not Satisfy." *American Journal of Clinical Nutrition* 62 (1995): 1–9.

Hibbeln, J. R., J. C. Umhau, D. T. George, and N. Salem Jr. *Do Plasma Polyunsaturates Predict Hostility and Violence? In Nutrition and Fitness: Metabolic and Behavior Aspects in Health and Disease, World Review of Nutrition and Dietetics.* Edited by A. P. Simopoulos and K. N. Pavlou. Basel, Switzerland: Karger, 1996, 175–86.

Holick, M. F. "Vitamin D Deficiency." *New England Journal of Medicine* 357 (2007): 266–81.

Holmes, M. D., D. J. Hunter, G. A. Colditz, et al. "Association of Dietary Intake of Fat and Fatty Acids with Risk of Breast Cancer." *Journal of the American Medical Association* 281 (1999): 914–20.

Hopkins, P. N. "Effects of Dietary Cholesterol on Serum Cholesterol: A Meta-Analysis and Review." *American Journal of Clinical Nutrition* 55 (1992): 1060–70.

Hsiao, P. J., K. K. Kuo, S. J. Shin, et al. "Significant Correlations between Severe Fatty Liver and Risk Factors for Metabolic Syndrome." *Journal of Gastroenterology and Hepatology* 22 (2007): 2118–23.

Hu, J., C. La Vecchia, L. Gibbons, et al. "Nutrients and Risk of Prostate Cancer." *Nutrition and Cancer* 62 (2010): 710–18.

Iribarrne, C., J. H. Markovitz, D. R. Jacobs, et al. "Dietary Intake of N-3, N-6 Fatty Acids and Fish: Relationship with Hostility in Young Adults—the CARDIA Study." *European Journal of Clinical Nutrition* 58 (2004): 24–31.

Iso, H., M. Kobayashi, J. Ishihara, et al. "Intake of Fish and N-3 Fatty Acids and Risk of Coronary Heart Disease among Japanese: The Japan Public Health Center-Bases (JPHC) Study Cohort I." *Circulation* 113 (2006): 195–202.

Itariu, B. K., Z. Maximillian, L. Leitner, et al. "Treatment with N-3 Polyunsaturated Fatty Acids Overcomes the Inverse Association of Vitamin D Deficiency with Inflammation in Severely Obese Patients: A Randomized Controlled Trial." *PLoS ONE* 8 (2013): e54634.

Iwata, N. G., M. Pham, N. O. Rizzo, et al. "Trans-Fatty Acids Induce Vascular Inflammation and Reduce Vascular Nitric Oxide Production in Endothelial Cells." *PloS ONE* 6 (2011):e29600.

Jacobs, E. J., C. C. Newton, Y. Wang, et al. "Waist Circumference and All-Cause Mortality in a Large US Cohort." *Archives of Internal Medicine* 170 (2010): 1293–301.

Jalal, D. I., G. Smits, and R. J. Johnson. "Increased Fructose Associates with Elevated Blood Pressure." *Journal of the American Society of Nephrology* 21 (2010): 1543–49.

Jenkins D. J., J. M. Wong, C. W. Kendall, et al. "The Effect of a Plant-Based Low-Carbohydrate ('Eco-Atkins') Diet on Body Weight and Blood Lipid Concentrations in Hyperlipidemic Subjects." *Archives of Internal Medicine* 169 (2009): 1046–54.

Johnson, R. J., T. Nakagawa, L. G. Sanchez-Lozada, et al. "Sugar, Uric Acid, and the Etiology of Diabetes and Obesity." *Diabetes* 62 (2013): 3307–15.

Johnston, B. C., S. Kanters, K. Bandayrel, et al. "Comparison of Weight Loss among Named Diet Programs in Overweight and Obese Adults: A Meta-Analysis." *Journal of the American Medical Association* 312 (2014): 923–33.

Johnston, P. V., O. C. Johnson, and F. A. Kummerow. "Occurrence of Trans-Fatty Acids in Human Tissue." *Science* 126 (1957): 698–99.

Judd, J. T., B. A. Clevidence, R. A. Muesing, et al. "Dietary Trans-Fatty Acids: Effects on Plasma Lipids and Lipoproteins of Healthy Men and Women." *American Journal of Clinical Nutrition* 59 (1994): 861–68.

Kalogeropoulos, N., D. B. Panagiotakos, C. Pitsavos, et al. "Unsaturated Fatty Acids Are Inversely Associated, and N-6/N-3 Ratios Are Positively Related to Inflammation and Coagulation Mrkders in Plasma in Apparently Healthy Adults." *Clinica Chimica Acta* 411 (2010): 584–91.

Kang, J. X. "Differential Effects of Omega-6 and Omega-3 Fatty Acids on Telomere Length." *American Journal of Clinical Nutrition* 92 (2010): 1276–77.

Kaplan, R. M., and M. T. Toshima. "Does a Reduced Fat Diet Cause Retardation in Child Growth?" *Preventive Medicine* 21 (1992): 33–52.

Kark, J. D., A. H. Smith, and C. G. Hames. "The Relationship of Serum Cholesterol to the Incidence of Cancer in Evans County, Georgia." *Journal of Chronic Diseases* 33 (1980): 311–22.

Kelishadi, R., M. Mansourian, and M. Heidari-Beni. "Association of Fructose Consumption and Components of Metabolic Syndrome in Human Studies: A Systemic Review and Meta-Analysis." *Nutrition* 30 (2014): 503–10.

Kelleher, P. C., S. D. Phinney, E. A. H. Sims, et al. "Effects of Carbohydrate-Containing and Carbohydrate-Restricted Hypocaloric and Eucaloric Diets on Serum Concentrations of Retinol-Binding Protein, Thyroxine-Binding Prealbumin and Transferrin." *Metabolism* 32 (1983): 95–101.

Kern, F. "Normal Cholesterol in an 88-Year-Old Man Who Eats 25 Eggs a Day: Mechanisms of Adaptation." *New England Journal of Medicine* 324 (1991): 896–99.

Key, T. J., P. N. Appleby, E. A. Spencer, R. C. Travis, et al. "Mortality in British Vegetarians: Results from the European Prospective Investigation into Cancer and Nutrition." *American Journal of Clinical Nutrition* 89 (2009): 1613s–1619s.

Keys, A. "Diet and the Epidemiology of Coronary Heart Disease." *Journal of the American Medical Association* 164 (1957): 1912–19.

Kiage, J. N., P. D. Merrill, C. J. Robinson, et al. "Intake of Trans Fat and All-Cause Mortality in the Reasons for Geographical and Racial Differences in Stroke (REGARDS) Cohort." *American Journal of Clinical Nutrition* 97 (2013): 1121–28.

Kiecolt-Glaser, J. K., M. A. Belury, R. Andridge, et al. "Omega-3 Supplementation Lowers Inflammation and Anxiety in Medical Students: A Randomized Controlled Trial." *Brain Behavior and Immunity* 25 (2011): 1725–34.

Kiecolt-Glaser, J. K., M. A. Belury, R. Andridge, et al. "Omega-3 Supplementation Lowers Inflammation in Healthy Middle-Aged and Older Adults: A Randomized Controlled Trial." *Brain Behavior and Immunity* 26 (2012): 988–95.

Kiecolt-Glaser, J. K., E. S. Epel, M. A. Belury, et al. "Omega-3 Fatty Acids, Oxidative Stress, and Leukocyte Telomere Length: A Randomized Controlled Trial." *Brain Behavior and Immunity* 28 (2013): 16–24.

Kneepkens, C. M., R. J. Vonk, and J. Fernandes. "Incomplete Intestinal Absorption of Fructose." *Archives of Diseases of Children* 59 (1984): 735–38.

Knopp, R. H., P. Paramsothy, B. M. Retzlaff, et al. "Gender Differences in Lipoprotein Metabolism and Dietary Response: Basis in Hormonal Differences and Implications for Cardiovascular Disease." *Current Atherosclerosis Reports* 7 (2005): 472–79.

Knopp, R. H., B. Retzlaff, C. Walden, et al. "One-Year Effects of Increasingly Fat-Restricted, Carbohydrate-Enriched Diets on Lipoprotein Levels in Free-Living Subjects." *Proceedings for the Society of Experimental Biology and Medicine* 225 (2000): 191–99.

Kozarevic, D., D. L. McGee, N. Vojvodic, et al. "Serum Cholesterol and Mortality: The Yugoslavia Cardiovascular Disease Study." *American Journal of Epidemiology* 114 (1981): 21–28.

Krauss, R. M. "Dietary and Genetic Probes of Atherogenic Dyslipidemia." *Arteriosclerosis, Thrombosis, and Vascular Biology* 25 (2005): 2265–72.

Krauss, R. M., P. J. Blanche, R. S. Rawlings, et al. "Separate Effects of Reduced Carbohydrate Intake and Weight Loss on Atherogenic Dyslipidemia." *American Journal of Clinical Nutrition* 83 (2006): 1025–31.

Kraus R. M., and D. M. Dreon. "Low-Density-Lipoprotein Subclasses and Response to a Low-Fat Diet in Healthy Men." *American Journal of Clinical Nutrition* 62 (1995): 478S–487S.

Krauss, R. M., R. H. Eckel, B. Howard, et al. "AHA Dietary Guidelines Revision 2000: A Statement for Health Care Professionals from the Nutrition Committee of the American Heart Association." *Circulation* 102 (2000): 2284–99.

Kris-Etherton, P. M., M. Lefevre, R. P. Mensink, et al. "Trans-Fatty Acid Intakes and Food Sources in the US Population: NHANES 1999–2002." *Lipids* 47 (2012): 931–40.

Kromhout, D., A. Menotti, B. Bloemberg, et al. "Dietary Saturated and Trans-Fatty Acids and Cholesterol and 25-Year Mortality from Coronary Heart Disease: The Seven Countries Study." *Preventive Medicine* 24 (1995): 308–15.

Kuipers, R. et al. "Saturated Fat, Carbohydrates, and Cardiovascular Disease." *Netherlands Journal of Medicine* 69 (2011): 372–372.

Kummerow, F. A., T. Mizuguchi, T. Arima, et al. "The Influence of Three Sources of Dietary Fats and Cholesterol on Lipid Composition of Swine Lipids and Aorta Tissue." *Artery* 4 (1978): 360–84.

Kummerow, F. A., S. Q. Zhour, and M. M. Mahfouz. "Effects of Trans-Fatty Acids on Calcium Influx into Human Arterial Endothelial Cells." *American Journal of Clinical Nutrition* 70 (1999): 832–38.

Lavie, C. J., J. H. Lee, and R. V. Milani. "Vitamin D and Cardiovascular Disease." *Journal of the American College of Cardiology* 58 (2011): 1547–56.

Lavie, C. J., R. V. Milani, M. R. Mehra, and H. O. Ventura. "Omega-3 Polyunsaturated Fatty Acids and Cardiovascular Diseases." *Journal of the American College of Cardiology* 54 (2009): 585–94.

Lee J. H., J. H. O'Keefe, C. J. Lavie, and W. S. Harris. "Omega-3 Fatty Acids: Cardiovascular Benefits, Sources, and Sustainability." *Nature Reviews Cardiology* 6 (2009): 753–58.

Lemaitre, R. N., I. B. King, T. E. Raghunathan, et al. "Cell Membrane Trans-Fatty Acids and the Risk of Primary Cardiac Arrest." *Circulation* 105 (2002): 697–701.

Lichtenstein, A. H., L. J. Appel, M. Brands, et al. "Diet and Lifestyle Recommendation: A Scientific Statement From the American Heart Association Nutrition Committee." *Circulation* 114(2006): 82-96.

Lichtenstein, A. H., L. M. Ausman, W. Carrasco, et al. "Hydrogenation Impairs the Hypolipidemic Effect of Corn Oil in Humans. Hydrogenation, Trans-Fatty Acids, and Plasma Lipids." *Arteriosclerosis, Thrombosis, and Vascular Biology* 13 (1993): 154–61.

Lichtenstein, A. H., and L. Van Horn. "Very Low-Fat Diets." *Circulation* 98 (1998): 935–39.

Lin, C., Chang C., C. Lu, et al. "Impact of the Gut Microbiota, Prebiotics, and Probiotics on Human Health and Disease." *Biomedical Journal* 37 (2014): 259–68.

Lopez-Garcia, E., M. B. Schulze, J. B. Meigs, et al. "Consumption of Trans-Fatty Acids Is Related to Plasma Biomarkers of Inflammation and Endothelial Dysfunction." *Journal of Nutrition* 135 (2005): 562–66.

Lucas, R. M., S. Gorman, S. Geldenhuys, and P. H. Hart. "Vitamin D and Immunity." *F1000Prime Report* 6 (2014): 118, doi:10.127.

Lyons, M. F. *42 Days to a New Life*. Florida, Xulon Press, 2007.

Lyons, M. F. *Fructose Exposed*. Florida, Xulon Press, 2010.

Ma, Y., C. Yu, Z. Shen, et al. "Effects of Probiotics on Nonalcoholic Fatty Liver Disease: A Meta-Analysis." *World Journal of Gastroenterology* 19 (2013): 6911–18.

Marchioli, R., F. Barzi, E. Bomba, et al. "Early Protection against Sudden Death by N-3 Polyunsaturated Fatty Acids after Myocardial Infarction-Time Course Analysis of the Results of the Gruppo Italiano per lo Studio della Sopravvivennza nell'Infarto Miocarico (GISSI)-Prevenzione." *Circulation* 105 (2002): 1897–902.

Mattson, F. H., and S. M. Grundy. "Comparison of Effects of Dietary Saturated, Unsaturated, and Polyunsaturated Fatty Acids on Plasma Lipids and in Man." *Journal of Lipid Research* 26 (1985): 194–202.

McClernon, F. J., W. S. Yancy, J. A. Eberstein, R. C. Atkins, and E. C. Westman. "The Effects of a Low-Carbohydrate Ketogenic Diet and a Low-Fat Diet on Mood, Hunger, and Other Self-Reported Symptoms." *Obesity* 15 (2007): 182–87.

McOsker, D. E., F. H. Mattson, H. B. Sweringen, and A. M. Kligman. "The Influence of Partially Hydrogenated Dietary Fats on Serum Cholesterol Levels." *Journal of the American Medical Association* 180 (1962): 380–85.

Mensink, R. P., and M. B. Katan. "Effect of Dietary Trans-Fatty Acids on High-Density and Low-Density Lipoprotein Cholesterol Levels in Healthy Subjects." *New England Journal of Medicine* 323 (1990): 439–45.

Mensink, R. P., P. L. Zock, A. D. Kester, and M. B. Katan. "Effects of Dietary Fatty Acids and Carbohydrates on the Ratio of Serum Total to HDL Cholesterol and on Serum Lipids and Apolipoproteins: A Meta-Analysis of 60 Controlled Trials." *American Journal of Clinical Nutrition* 77 (2003): 1146–55.

Merritt, M. A., D. W. Cramer, S. A. Missmer, et al. "Dietary Fat Intake and Risk of Epithelial Ovarian Cancer by Tumour Histology." *British Journal of Cancer* 110 (2014): 1392–401.

Michels, K., and F. Sacks. "Trans-Fatty Acids in European Margarines." *New England Journal of Medicine* 332 (1995): 541–42.

Miller, S. R., P. I. Tartter, A. E. Papatestas, et al. "Serum Cholesterol and Human Colon Cancer." *Journal of the National Cancer Institute* 67 (1981): 297–300.

Minger, D. *Death by Food Pyramid*. Malibu, CA: Primal Blueprint, 2013.

Miyashita, Y., N. Koide, M. Ohtsuka, et al. "Beneficial Effect of Low Carbohydrate in Low-Calorie Diets on Visceral Fat Reduction in Type 2 Diabetic Patients with Obesity." *Diabetes Research and Clinical Practice* 65 (2004): 235–41.

Mozaffarian, D. "The Great Fat Debate: Taking the Focus off Saturated Fat." *Journal of the American Dietetic Association* 111 (2011): 665–66.

Mozaffarian, D., M. B. Katan, A. Ascherio, et al. "Trans-Fatty Acids and Cardiovascular Disease." *New England Journal of Medicine* 354 (2006): 1601–13.

Muldoon, M. F., S. B. Manuck, and K. A. Matthews. "Lowering Cholesterol Concentration and Mortality: A Quantitative Review of Primary Prevention Trials." *British Medical Journal* 301 (1990): 309–14.

Nestel, P. J., and A. Poyser. "Changes in Cholesterol Synthesis and Excretion When Cholesterol Intake Is Increased." *Metabolism* 25 (1976): 1591–99.

Neuschwander-Tetri, B. A. "Carbohydrate Intake and Nonalcoholic Fatty Liver Disease." *Current Opinion in Clinical Nutrition and Metabolic Care* 16 (2013): 446–52.

Nielsen, J. V., E. Jonsson, and A. K. Nilsson. "Lasting Improvement of Hyperglycaemia and Body Weight: Low-Carbohydrate Diet in Type 2 Diabetes. A Brief Report." *Upsala Journal of Medical Science* 110 (2005): 179–83.

Niramitmahapanya, S., S. S. Harris, and B. Dawson-Hughes. "Type of Dietary Fat Is Associated with the 25-Hydroxyvitamin D3 Increment in Response to Vitamin D Supplementation." *Journal of Clinical Endocrinology and Metabolism* 96 (2011): 3170–74.

Noakes, T. D. "The Women's Health Initiative Randomized Controlled Dietary Modification Trial: An Inconvenient Finding and the Diet-Heart Hypothesis." *South African Medical Journal* 103 (2013): 824–825.

Nordmann, A. J., A. Nordmann, M. Briel, et al. "Effects of Low-Carbohydrate vs. Low-Fat Diets on Weight Loss and Cardiovascular

Risk Factors: A Meta-Analysis of Randomized Controlled Trials." *Archives of Internal Medicine* 166 (2006): 285–93.

Nydegger, U. E., and R. E. Butler. "Serum Lipoprotein Levels in Patients with Cancer." *Cancer Research* 32 (1972): 1756–60.

Pan, A., D. Yu, W. Demark-Wahnefried, et al. "Meta-Analysis of the Effects of Flaxseed Interventions on Blood Lipids." *American Journal of Clinical Nutrition* 90 (2009): 288–97.

Pandey, V., V. Berwal, N. Solanki, and N. S. Malik. "Probiotics: Healthy Bugs and Nourishing Elements of Diet." *Journal of International Society of Preventive and Community Dentistry* 5 (2015): 81–87.

Park S., and J. H. Bae. "Probiotics for Weight Loss: A Systematic Review and Meta-Analysis." *Nutrition Research* (May 21, 2015), pii:S0271-5317(15)0000103-7, doi:10.1016/j.nutres.2015.05.008.

Patek, A. J., F. E. Kendall, N. M. De Fritsch, and R. L. Hirsch. "Cirrhosis-Enhancing Effect of Corn Oil." *Archives of Pathology* 82 (1966): 596–601.

Pearce, M. L., and S. Dayton. "Incidence of Cancer in Men on a Diet High in Polyunsaturated Fat." *Lancet* 297 (1971): 464–67.

Pehl, C., A. Pfeiffer, A. Waizenfoefer, B. Wendl, and W. Schepp. "Effect of Caloric Density of a Meal on Lower Oesophageal Sphincter Motility and Gastroesophageal Reflux in Healthy Subjects." *Alimentary Pharmacology and Therapeutics* 15 (2001): 233–39.

Pehl, C., A. Waizenhoefer, B. Wendl, et al. "Effect of Low and High Fat Meals on Lower Esophageal Sphincter Motility and Gastroesophageal

Reflux in Health Subjects." *American Journal of Gastroenterology* 94 (1999): 1192–96.

Pennington, A. W. "A Reorientation on Obesity." *New England Journal of Medicine* 248 (1953): 959–64.

Phinney, S. D., B. R. Bistrian, R. R. Wolfe, and G. L. Blackburn. "The Human Metabolic Response to Chronic Ketosis without Caloric Restriction: Physical and Biochemical Adaption." *Metabolism* 32 (1983): 757–68.

Phinney, S. D., E. S. Horton, E. A. H. Sims, et al. "Capacity for Moderate Exercise in Obese Subjects after Adaptation to a Hypocaloric, Ketogenic Diet." *Journal of Clinical Investigation* 66 (1980): 1152–61.

Piche, T., S. B. des Varannes, S. Sacher-Huvelin, et al. "Colonic Fermentation Influences Lower Esophageal Sphincter Function in Gastroesophageal Reflux Disease." *Gastroenterology* 124 (2003): 894–902.

Pinckney, E. R., and C. Pinckey. *The Cholesterol Controversy.* Los Angeles: Sherbourne Press, 1973.

Pottala, J. V., S. Garg, B. E. Cohen, et al. "Blood Eicosapentaenoic and Docosaheaenoic Acids Predict All-Cause Mortality in Patients with Stable Coronary Heart Disease: The Heart and Soul Study." *Circulation: Cardiovascular Quality and Outcomes* 3 (2010): 406–12.

Poustie, V. J., and P. Rutherford. "Dietary Treatment for Familial Hypercholesterolemia." *Cochrane Database of Systematic Reviews* 2 (2001): CD001918.

Prior, I. A., F. Davidson, C. E. Salmond, and Z. Czochanska. "Cholesterol, Coconuts, and Diet on Polynesian Atolls: A Natural Experiment: The Pukapuka and Tokelau Island Studies." *American Journal of Clinical Nutrition* 34 (1981): 1552–61.

Qintao, E., S. Grundy, and E. H. Ahrens Jr. "Effects of Dietary Cholesterol on the Regulation of Total Body Cholesterol in Man." *Journal of Lipid Research* 12 (1971): 233–47.

Raimundo, F. V., G. A. M. Faulhaber, P. K. Menegatti, et al. "Effect of High- versus Low-Fat Meal on Serum 25-Hydroxyvitamin D Levels after a Single Oral Dose of Vitamin D: A Single-Blind, Parallel, Randomized Trial." *International Journal of Endocrinology*, 2011, doi:10.1155/2011/809609.

Ramsden, C. E., J. R. Hibbeln, S. F. Majchrzak, and J. M. Davis. "N-6 Fatty Acid-Specific and Mixed Polyunsaturate Dietary Interventions Have Different Effects on CHD Risk: A Meta-Analysis of Randomized Controlled Trials." *British Journal of Nutrition* 104 (2010): 1586–600.

Rand, M. L., A. A. Hennissen, and G. Hornstra. "Effects of Dietary Palm Oil on Arterial Thrombosis, Platelet Responses, and Platelet Membrane Fluidity in Rats." *Lipids* 23 (1988): 1019–23.

Ravich, W. J., T. M. Bayless, and M. Thomas. "Fructose: Incomplete Intestinal Absorption in Humans." *Gastroenterology* 84 (1983): 26–29.

Ravnskov, U. *The Cholesterol Myths: Exposing the Fallacy That Saturated Fat and Cholesterol Cause Heart Disease.* Washington, DC: New Trends, 2000.

Razmpoosh, E., M. Javadi, H. S. Ejtahed, and P. Mirmiran. "Probiotics as Beneficial Agents in the Management of Diabetes Mellitus: A Systematic Review." *Diabetes/Metabolism Research Reviews* (May 11, 2015), doi:10.1002/dmrr.2665.

Reiser, S., A. S. Powell, D. J. Scholfield, et al. "Blood Lipids, Lipoproteins, Apoproteins, and Uric Acid in Men Fed Diets Containing Fructose or High-Amylose Cornstarch." *American Journal of Clinical Nutrition* 49 (1989): 832–39.

Rivellese, A. A., R. Giacco, G. Annuzzi, et al. "Effects of Monosaturated vs. Saturated Fat on Postprandial Lipemia and Adipose Tissue Lipases in Type 2 Diabetes." *Clinical Nutrition* 27 (2008): 133–41.

Riveros, M. J., A. Parada, and P. Pettinelli. "Fructose Consumption and Its Health Implications: Fructose Malabsorption and Nonalcoholic Fatty Liver Disease." *Nutricion Hospitalaria* 29 (2014): 491–99.

Rogers, A. E., and M. P. Longnecker. "Biology of Disease: Dietary and Nutritional Influences on Cancer: A Review of Epidemiological and Experimental Data." *Laboratory Investigation* 59 (1988): 729–59.

Rong, Y., L. Chen, T. Zhu, et al. Egg Consumption and Risk of Coronary Heart Disease and Stroke: dose-Response Meta-Analysis of Prospective Cohort Studies. British Medical Journal 346 (2013): e8539.

Rose, G., H. Blackburn, A. Keys, et al. "Colon Cancer and Blood-Cholesterol." *Lancet* 303 (1974): 181–83.

Ruan, Y., J. Sun, J. He, et al. "Effect of Probiotics on Glycemic Control: A Systematic Review and Meta-Analysis of Randomized, Controlled Trials." *Plos One*, July 10, 2015, doi:10.1371/journal.pone.0132121.

Sacks, F. M., G. A. Bray, V. J. Carey, et al. "Comparison of Weight-Loss Diets with Different Compositions of Fat, Protein, and Carbohydrates." *New England Journal of Medicine* 360 (2009): 859–73.

Sacks, F. M., and L. Litlin. "Trans-Fatty Acid Content of Common Foods." *New England Journal of Medicine* 329 (1993): 1969–70.

Samaha, F. F., N. Iqbal, P. Seshadri, et al. "A Low-Carbohydrate as Compared with a Low-Fat Diet in Severe Obesity." *New England Journal of Medicine* 348 (2003): 2074–81.

Sargrad, K. R., C. Homko, M. Mozzoli, and G. Boden. "Effect of High-Protein vs High-Carbohydrate Intake on Insulin Sensitivity, Body Weight, Hemoglobin A1c, and Blood Pressure in Patients with Type 2 Diabetes Mellitus." *Journal of the American Dietetic Association* 105 (2005): 573–80.

Schleifer, D. "We Spent a Million Bucks, and Then We Had to Do Something: The Unexpected Implications of Industry Involvement in Trans Fat Research." *Bulletin of Science, Technology, and Society* 31 (2011): 460–71.

Schmid, A., and B. Walther. "Natural Vitamin D Content in Animal Products." *Advances in Nutrition* 4 (2013): 453–62.

Sekikawa, A., J. D. Curb, H. Ueshima, et al. "Marine-Derived N-3 Fatty Acids and Atherosclerosis in Japanese, Japanese-American and White Men." *Journal of the American College of Cardiology* 52 (2008): 417–24.

Serra-Majem, L., L. Ribas, R. Tresserras, J. Ngo, and L. Salleras. "How Could Changes in Diet Explain Changes in Coronary Heart Disease

Mortality in Spain? The Spanish Paradox." *American Journal of Clinical Nutrition* 61 (1995): 1351S–1359S.

Shai, I., D. Schwarzfuch, Y. Henkin, et al. "Weight Loss with a Low-Carbohydrate, Mediterranean, or Low-Fat Diet." *New England Journal of Medicine* 359 (2008): 229–41.

Sharman, M. J., A. L. Gomez, W. J. Kraemer, and J. S. Volek. "Very Low-Carbohydrate and Low-Fat Diets Affect Fasting Lipids and Postprandial Lipemia Differently in Overweight Men." *Journal of Nutrition* 134 (2004): 880–85.

Shaw, J. *Trans Fats: The Hidden Killer in our Food.* New York: Pocket Books, 2004.

Shin, J. Y., J. Suls, and R. Martin. "Are Cholesterol and Depression Inversely Related? A Meta-Analysis of the Association between Two Cardiac Risk Factors." *Annals of Behavioral Medicine* 36 (2008): 33–43.

Siguel, E. N., and R. H. Lerman. "Role of Essential Fatty Acids: Dangers in the US Department of Agriculture Dietary Recommendations ('Pyramid') and in Low-Fat Diets." *American Journal of Clinical Nutrition* 60 (1994): 973–74.

Simopoulos A. P. "The Importance of the Omega-6/Omega-3 Fatty Acid Ratio in Cardiovascular Disease and Other Chronic Diseases." *Experimental Biology and Medicine* 233 (2008): 674–88.

Siri-Tarino, P. W., Q. Sun, F. B. Hu, and R. M. Krauss. "Saturated Fat, Carbohydrates, and Cardiovascular Disease." *American Journal of Clinical Nutrition* 91 (2010): 502–9.

Smit, L. A., M. B. Katan, A. J. Wanders, et al. "A High Intake of Trans-Fatty Acids Has Little Effect on Markers of Inflammation and Oxidative Stress in Humans". *Journal of Nutrition* 141 (2011): 1673–78.

Stanhope, K. L., J. M. Schwartz, N. L. Keim, et al. "Consuming Fructose-Sweetened, Not Glucose-Sweetened, Beverages Increases Visceral Adiposity and Lipids and Decreases Insulin Sensitivity in Overweight/Obese Humans." *Journal of Clinical Investigation* 119 (2009): 1322–34.

Stemmermann, G. N., A. Nomura, L. K. Heilbrun, et al. "Serum Cholesterol and Colon Cancer Incidence in Hawaiian Japanese Men." *Journal of the National Cancer Institute* 67 (1981): 1179–82.

Stranges, S., J. M. Dorn, P. Muti, et al. "Body Fat Distribution, Relative Weight, and Liver Enzyme Levels: A Population-Based Study." *Hepatology* 39 (2004): 754–63.

Sun, B., and M. Karin. "Obesity, Inflammation, and Liver Cancer." *Journal of Hepatology* 56 (2012): 704–13.

Sun, Q., J. Ma, H. Campos, et al. "A Prospective Study of Trans-Fatty Acids in Erythrocytes and Risk of Coronary Heart Disease." *Circulation* 115 (2007): 1858–65.

Sun, Q., J. Ma, H. Campos, et al. "Comparison between Plasma and Erythrocyte Fatty Acid Content as Biomarkers of Fatty Acid Intake in US Women." *American Journal of Clinical Nutrition* 86 (2007): 74–81.

Tarantino, G., and C. Finelli. "Systematic Review on Intervention with Prebiotics/Probiotics in Patients with Obesity-Related Nonalcoholic Fatty Liver Disease." *Future Microbiology* 10 (2015): 889–902.

Taubes, G.. "The Soft Science of Dietary Fat." *Science* 291 (2001): 2536–45.

Teicholz, N. *The Big Fat Surprise: Why Butter, Meat, and Cheese Belong in a Healthy Diet.* New York: Simon and Schuster, 2014.

Usai, P., R. Manca, R. Cuomo, et al. "Effect of Gluten-Free Diet on Preventing Recurrence of Gastroesophageal Reflux Disease-Related Symptoms in Adult Celiac Patients with Nonerosive Reflux Disease." *Journal of Gastroenterology and Hepatology* 23 (2008): 1368–72.

Van Deventer, H., W. G. Miller, G. L. Meyers, et al. "Non-HDL Cholesterol Shows Improved Accuracy for Cardiovascular Risk Score Classification Compared to Direct or Calculated LDL Cholesterol in Dyslipidemic Population." *Clinical Chemistry* 57 (2011): 490–501.

Vinikoor, L. C., J. C. Schroeder, R. C. Millikan, et al. "Consumption of Trans-Fatty Acid and Its Association with Colorectal Adenomas." *American Journal of Epidemiology* 168 (2008): 289–97.

Volek J. S., K. D. Ballard, R. Silvestre, et al. "Effects of Dietary Carbohydrate Restriction vs. Low-Fat Diet on Flow-Mediated Dilation." *Metabolism* 58 (2009): 1769–77.

Volek, J. S., S. D. Phinney, C. E. Forsythe, et al. "Carbohydrate Restriction Has a More Favorable Impact on the Metabolic Syndrome Than a Low-Fat Diet. *Lipids* 44 (2009): 297–309.

Volek, J. S., M. J. Sharman, et al. "Comparison of a Very Low-Carbohydrate and Low-Fat Diet on Fasting Lipids, LDL Subclasses, Insulin Resistance, and Postprandial Lipemic Responses in Overweight

Women." *Journal of the American College of Nutrition* 23 (2004): 177–84.

Vos, M. B., J. E. Lavine. "Dietary Fructose in Nonalcoholic Fatty Liver Disease." *Hepatology* 57 (2013): 2525–31.

Westman, E. C. "Rethinking Dietary Saturated Fat." *Food Technology* 63 (2009): 30.

Westman, E. C., R. D. Feinman, J. C. Mavropoulos, et al. "Low-Carbohydrate Nutrition and Metabolism." *American Journal of Clinical Nutrition* 86 (2007): 276–84.

Westman, E. C., J. S. Volek, and R. D. Feinman. "Carbohydrate Restriction Is Effective in Improving Dyslipidemia Even in the Absence of Weight Loss." *American Journal of Clinical Nutrition* 84 (2006): 1549.

Westman, E. C., W. S. Yancy, J. S. Edman, et al. "Effect of 6-Month Adherence to a Very Low-Carbohydrate Diet Program." *American Journal of Medicine* 113 (2002): 30–36.

Willett, W. C., and D. J. Hunter. "Prospective Studies of Diet and Breast Cancer." *Cancer* 74 (1994): 1085–89.

Willett, W. C, M. J. Stampfer, G. A. Colditz, et al. "Dietary Fat and the Risk of Breast Cancer." *New England Journal of Medicine* 316 (1987): 22–28.

Willett, W. C., M. J. Stampfer, J. E. Manson, et al. "Intake of Trans-Fatty Acids and Risk of Coronary Heart Disease among Women." *Lancet* 341 (1993): 581–85.

Williams, R. R., P. D. Sorlie, M. Feinleib, et al. "Cancer Incidence by Levels of Cholesterol." *Journal of the American Medical Association* 245 (1981): 247–52.

Wolfe, L. *Eat the Yolks.* Nevada, Victory Belt, 2013.

Wood, R., F. Chumbler, and R. Wiegand. "Incorporation of Dietary Cis and Trans Isomers of Octadecenoate in Lipid Classes of Liver and Hepatoma." *Journal of Biological Chemistry* 252 (1977): 1965–70.

Wood, R., K. Kubena, B. O'Brien, et al. "Effect of Butter, Mono-, and Polyunsaturated Fatty Acid-Enriched Butter, Trans-Fatty Acid Margarine, and Zero Trans-Fatty Acid Margarine on Serum Lipids and Lipoproteins in Healthy Men." *Journal of Lipid Research* 34 (1993): 1–11.

Wood R., K. Kubena, S. Tseng, et al. "Effect of Palm Oil, Margarine, Butter, and Sunflower Oil on Serum Lipids and Lipoproteins of Normocholesterolemic Middle-Aged Men." *Journal of Nutritional Biochemistry* 4 (1993): 286–97.

www.mayoclinic.org/diseases-conditions/gerd/basics/symptoms/con-20025201. Accessed 7/10/2015.

www.niddk.nih.gov/health-information/health-topics/digestive-diseases/ger-and-gerd. Accessed 7/10/2015.

www.nutritiondat.self.com/facts. Nutrition Facts about Salmon and Beef. Accessed 8/13/2015.

www.webmd.com/heartburn-gerd/guide/reflux-disease-gerd-1. Accessed 7/10/2015.

Yaemsiri, S., S. Sen, L. Tinker, et al. "Trans Fat, Aspirin, and Ischemic Stroke in Postmenopausal Women." *Annals of Neurology* 72 (2012): 704–15.

Yam, D., A. Eliraz, and E. M. Berry. "Diet and Disease—The Israeli Paradox: Possible Dangers of a High Omega-6 Polyunsaturated Fatty Acid Diet." *Israel Journal of Medical Sciences* 32 (1996): 1134–43.

Yancy, W. S., M. K. Olsen, J. R. Guyton, et al. "A Low-Carbohydrate, Ketogenic Diet versus a Low-Fat Diet to Treat Obesity and Hyperlipidemia: A Randomized, Controlled Trial." *Annals of Internal Medicine* 140 (2004): 769–77.

Yancy, W. S., D. Provenzale, and E. C. Westman. "Improvement of Gastroesophageal Reflux Disease after Initiation of a Low-Carbohydrate Diet: Five Brief Case Reports." *Alternative Therapies in Health and Medicine* 7 (2001): 116–19.

Yang, B., X. Ren, Y. Fu, J. Gao, and L. Duo. "Ratio of N-3/N-6 PUFAs and Risk of Breast Cancer: A Meta-Analysis of 274,135 Adult Females from 11 Independent Prospective Studies." *BMC Cancer* 14 (2014): 105.

Yee, L. D., J. L. Lester, R. M. Cole, et al. "Omega-3 Fatty Acid Supplements in Women at High Risk of Breast Cancer Have Dose-Dependent Effects on Breast Adipose Tissue Fatty Acid Composition." *American Journal of Clinical Nutrition* 91 (2010): 1185–94.

Yokoyama, M., H. Origasa, M. Matsuzaki, et al. "Effects of Eicosapentaenoic Acid on Major Coronary Events in Hypercholesterolaemic Patients (JELIS): A Randomized, Open-Label, Blinded Endpoint Analysis." *Lancet* 369 (2007): 1090–98.

Zhang, M., W. Qian, Y. Qin, J. He, and Y. Zhou. "Probiotics in Helicobacter Pylori Eradication Therapy: A Systematic Review and Meta-Analysis." *World Journal of Gastroenterology* 21 (2015): 4345–57.

Zock, P. L., and M. B. Katan. "Hydrogenation Alternatives: Effects of Trans-Fatty Acids and Steric Acid vs. Linoleic Acid on Serum Lipids and Lipoproteins in Humans." *Journal of Lipid Research* 33 (1992): 399–410.